The Virtue of Patients:
Making
Best Use of Ward
Nursing Resources

LONDON: HMSO

©   *Crown copyright*

First published December 1991

ISBN 0 11 886 068 2

London : HMSO

Audit Commission, National Health Service Report No. 4

Printed by Honey Press Ltd. for the Audit Commission.

Preface

The Audit Commission became responsible for the external audit of the National Health Service (NHS) in October 1990. As well as reviewing the financial accounts of all Health Service bodies, the Commission's auditors have a duty to examine the economy, efficiency and effectiveness of health authorities' use of resources. Each year several health service topics or service areas are selected for special study.

The Commission's aim is to help those who manage and work in the NHS to deliver the best possible service within the expenditure level determined by Government. Sometimes this means finding ways of doing things more efficiently and cheaply, thus freeing resources which may be more effectively used elsewhere in the service. But cost-cutting is not an end in itself; the ultimate objective must be to ensure that NHS expenditure makes the maximum contribution to enhancing the health status of the population.

Often this contribution is difficult to define and measure. But in most areas there are measures of output and process efficiency which can be useful proxies for the eventual outcome. Nursing is a case in point. This is the first Audit Commission study to concentrate on the management of **ward nursing in acute general hospitals**. The detailed work of the study was conducted on general medical, general surgical and acute care of the elderly wards, but many of the findings and recommendations have broader application.

In addition to this report which gives an overview of the topic, the Commission will publish two further papers targeted at those directly involved in managing wards and nursing services, one on improving patient care on acute general wards, the other on the effective use of nurse management systems.

The project team looked in detail at 39 wards in 10 NHS hospitals chosen to provide a geographical cross-section, a variety of sizes, nurse management structures and systems and approaches to promoting quality of care. It also paid brief visits to other NHS and private hospitals in this country, and to hospitals in France and the USA to explore specific developments in nursing management or organisation of care. The team has been advised periodically during the course of the study by a panel of senior nurses, managers and academics and by a group of ward sisters and clinical nurse managers. The Commission is grateful to the many organisations and individuals who have offered comments. A list of contacts and team members is given at appendix 1.

In parallel with the publication of this report, auditors will begin reviews of nursing in selected wards and hospitals drawn from each health authority and trust. These reviews will produce specific recommendations tailored to local circumstances and constraints. Their scope and methodology is described in a separate Audit Guide to be published shortly.

Table of Contents

SUMMARY   1

INTRODUCTION   3
— Changing Inpatient Needs   3
— Lack of Knowledge about Outcomes: 4
— What is the Role of the Nurse?   4
— Project 2000.   6
— What Constitutes 'Good' Nursing?   7
— How this Report can Help   8

1. DELIVERING BETTER PATIENT CARE   11
— Measuring Quality to Improve Care   11
— Quality Assurance   14
— Making care more Patient Centred   17
  Factors Inhibiting Patient Centred Care   18
  Are these Solutions Sufficient?   20
— Improving Continuity of Care   20
  How is Care Organised at Present?   21
  Why has Change become Necessary?   21
  Problems in Making Continuity of Care a Reality   23
  Improving Continuity of Care   25

2. STAFFING THE WARDS   27
— Problems in Determining how many Nurses are Needed?   27
  Lack of Research Linking Staffing to Outcomes   27
— Developing Clinical Skills   37
— Making best day-to-day use of Ward Staff   40

3. MANAGING THE NURSING SERVICE   49
— Styles of Management   49
— Systems   52
— Choosing an Appropriate Nursing Management Structure   54
— Strategy   57
  Implementing the Strategy   59

CONCLUSION   61
   — Summary of Recommendations   62
   — 1. Delivering Better Patient Care 62
   — 2. Staffing the wards   63
   — 3. Managing the nursing service   64

REFERENCES   67

APPENDIX 1   69
   — CONTACTS AND TEAM MEMBERS   69

GLOSSARY   73

Summary

Nursing is by far the largest item in a hospital's budget. It accounts for over a third of health authorities' revenue expenditure and almost half of their salary bills. Nurses also exercise effective control over much other hospital expenditure. General nursing on wards in acute hospitals, which is the focus of this report, costs some £1.2 billions per year.

Standards of nursing care are crucial to public perceptions of the quality of the National Health Service. Patients invariably say that nurses are wonderful, but there is increasing evidence that they would like more information about their treatment and care and a greater say in what happens to them in hospital.

Nursing in acute hospitals is facing a period of significant change for a number of reasons:

— **The inpatient population:** is older, frailer and in a less stable condition requiring skilled nursing.

— **The supply of nurses:** The decline in school leavers over the next few years and the rising career expectations of young women will challenge health authorities to improve the recruitment and retention of necessary skills.

— **Project 2000:** the biggest change to nursing education this century, has profound implications for staffing the wards.

— **Management:** changes arising out of the the NHS Reforms.

Constraints on the supply of skilled nurses and continuing pressure on resources mean that nursing skills must be deployed and managed as effectively as is possible if the quality of care is to improve. Evidence collected for the study suggests that some resources within nursing could be used more efficiently to release funds for investment in clinical training, and professional and managerial development for nurses. Hospitals vary significantly in the length of the overlap between morning and afternoon shifts, in the extent to which nurses perform clerical and housekeeping duties and in the costs of managing nursing. A reduction in the overlap to a maximum of one hour throughout the country could theoretically release resources of £50 million; reducing the proportion of nurses' time spent on non-nursing duties to eight per cent would release £ 40 million; whilst containing the costs of managing nursing services to no more than two percent of the nursing pay budget would release £35 million nationally for re-investment in services and training.

Nursing care needs to become more tailored to the needs of individual patients. There is also not enough continuity of care. Patients often do not know which nurse or group of nurses is looking after them, or who is able to give them information about their treatment. Many hospitals do not pay enough attention to assessing the quality of nursing, and in some, the effort put into improving quality goes to waste – either because senior managers have not established a framework for quality assurance, or because standards are not monitored once they have been set.

Nurses can only develop patient centred care if ward staffing reflects the needs of patients. In many hospitals at present there is no regular systematic review of ward establishments and a lack of consensus on patient care roles for unqualified staff. Many nurses still spend over a quarter of their time on clerical and housekeeping tasks. Large differences in the staffing of wards from day to day do not reflect workload. A minority of wards systematically collect data on nursing workload and fewer still put the resulting information to constructive use. Bank nurses are frequently booked regardless of predicted workload or the effect of large numbers of different 'temporary' staff on continuity of patient care.

Some wards show that it is possible, at little or no extra cost, to improve patient care and create more satisfying jobs for nurses. These are wards where the ward sister has actively used the duty roster and the method of allocating patients to nurses to promote continuity of patient-nurse relationships. Some sisters have used workload assessment to plan ahead. And, within the parameters of the budgets, nurse managers and ward sisters have used the authority delegated to them to change shifts and order temporary staff in ways that improve the match of staff to workload and protect continuity of patient care. Wards have made demonstrable improvements to standards of care by involving all their nurses in writing, monitoring and regularly reviewing standards. The advent of units in many hospitals, committed to the development and evaluation of nursing practice, is welcome.

Replicating these changes elsewhere will pose formidable challenges to general managers and nurse managers. There is a need for strong professional leadership of the nursing service. Nursing management structures need to be leaner and more clinically based, whilst retaining responsibilities for nursing advice at senior management level. In many hospitals there is room to improve staffing information and personnel practice and procedures. At all levels it is increasingly important to place the right nurse in the right job and provide her with support and opportunities for clinical and management development. Budgetary, patient information, nurse management and quality assessment systems need to be reviewed, and more attention paid to finding out patients' opinions in hospital.

Nursing is too important a component of patient care and of hospital budgets to be left to develop in isolation. The commitment of general managers and doctors in management, as well as managers of nursing services to an agreed vision and strategy for the development of nursing services is vital.

Introduction

1. Expenditure on nursing in the Hospital and Community Health Services of England and Wales was almost £ 5 billion in 1988-89. This was 36 per cent of health authorities' revenue expenditure and almost half of their salary bill. A quarter was spent on general nursing on adult acute wards in general hospitals (Exhibit 1). The management of that ward based nursing forms the principal subject of this report.

Exhibit 1
NHS PAY EXPENDITURE
Nursing accounts for almost half of   ...Over a quarter of nursing expenditure relates to
NHS Salaries...   adult acute wards

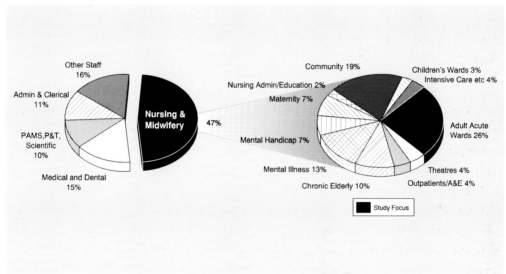

Source: Audit Commission estimates based on Health & PSS Statistics (England) and Department of Health Census of NHS Non-Medical Manpower: 30 Sept 1989

2. The Health Service Reforms place greater emphasis than ever before on cost-effective use of this major resource. There is more emphasis on critical review of staffing and grade-mix in relation to nursing workload and agreed standards. Hospitals are introducing new systems to cost the nursing care given to individual groups of patients so as to set contract prices and to monitor the quality of care that they provide against nursing care requirements specified in contracts.

CHANGING INPATIENT NEEDS

3. The average age of the inpatient population in all types of acute wards is rising. This is both because of general demographic trends and because a higher proportion of younger patients are now treated in day case units or as out-patients. Inpatients today are likely to be frailer and in need of greater nursing attention. In the past it was normal for some general medical and

---

*   *Note: Some 94 per cent of nurses working in areas considered by this report are women. For convenience therefore, the female pronoun and the term 'ward sister' are used throughout this report to refer to nursing staff. Patients, whether male or female, are referred to as "he".*

3

general surgical inpatients to be convalescent. Now most are only in hospital for the time that they are acutely ill. As a result, most inpatients are likely to be more dependent on skilled nursing care, and, because their condition is less stable, more in need of frequent monitoring by qualified nurses. The earlier discharge of patients from the hospital needs to be planned carefully. And qualified staff need time to prepare patients for their discharge and to teach those who are chronically ill how to cope with their symptoms at home.

LACK OF KNOWLEDGE ABOUT OUTCOMES:

4. The NHS Reforms increase the pressure to find outcome measures for nursing that will enable purchasers and providers to specify relationships between ward resources, the organisation of nursing care and quality. Health outcomes are notoriously difficult to measure, not least because it is rarely possible to separate out the contributions that the different professions make to the care of an individual patient. So, for example, whilst there is a distinct difference between patients' medical and nursing needs, a proportion of nurses' work with patients is carried out under doctors' orders and is determined by individual doctors' styles of clinical practice.

5. In the absence of reliable outcome measures for nursing, discussions about the quality of nursing services have tended to concentrate on the process of care and on organisational audit. The closest most contracts between purchasers and providers come to specifying the quality of nursing services has been to require hospitals to collect and supply information on, for example, drug administration errors, accidents and falls and to have systematic methods of quality assessment in place. The diversity of approaches to specifying quality in nursing will make it difficult for purchasers to compare the quality of service offered by hospitals within their areas with that of alternative providers.

WHAT IS THE ROLE OF THE NURSE?

6. There is ambiguity too about the role of the nurse in the acute hospital ward setting. According to Henderson's definition (Ref. 1):

> 'The unique function of the nurse is to assist the individual, sick or well, in the performance of those activities contributing to health or its recovery (or to peaceful death) that he would perform unaided if he had the necessary strength, will or knowledge. And to do this in such a way as to enable him to gain independence as rapidly as possible'.

7. A wide range of competencies are required by law to undertake this role (Ref. 2, Exhibit 2). But also, as noted in a recent King's Fund report, 'at different periods nurses have done (and do) work which could be considered the province of cleaners, dietitians, porters, clerks, secretaries, ward housekeepers, receptionists and doctors' (Ref. 3). Clinical advance has hastened the evolution of their role. Nurses in acute wards spend an increasing amount of time on tests and investigations and undertake sophisticated nursing interventions. In many hospitals, the nursing role has been extended to include tasks such as giving intravenous injections which were once the province of medical staff. The reduction in junior doctors' hours may bring pressure for further expansion in this direction, perhaps leading to the introduction of the 'super-nurse' (Ref. 4). And greater delegation of financial and personnel responsibilities to wards, hastened by the spread of clinical directorates, means that many nurses also have an increasing administrative role (Exhibit 3).

Exhibit 2
THE ROLE OF THE NURSE (1)
A wide range of competencies are required by law to undertake this role

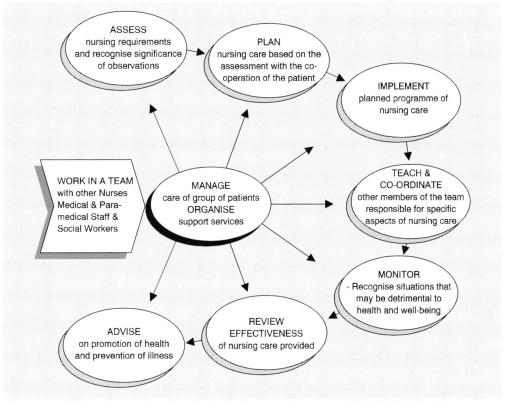

Source: Audit Commission. Based on Rule 18, Statutory Instrument 873 (1983) of the Act

Exhibit 3
THE ROLE OF THE NURSE (2)

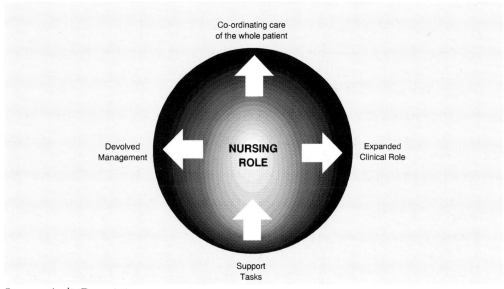

Source: Audit Commission.

8. More fundamentally, the drive to establish nursing as an independent profession has been marked by a greater emphasis on patient centred care. Today, nurses stress the importance for the patient's recovery of attending to his psychological and emotional needs, as well as his need for physical care. Surveys show that patients value personal contact with nurses. Specialisation in health care means that the number of professionals involved in the care of individual patients is increasing, both in hospital and in the community. Nurses have more contact with patients during their stay in hospital than do any other health professionals, and therefore more opportunity to get to know them personally. They are best placed to co-ordinate other professionals' work with the patient and, should the need arise, to represent the patient's interest at times when he is too ill, or lacks the ability or information to do so for himself, (Exhibit 4).

PROJECT 2000.

9. Implementation of Project 2000, the biggest change to nurse education this century, is likely to stimulate further changes. Under the traditional nursing apprenticeship system, 'learners' pick up many of their skills by working alongside nurses on wards. In practice, the pressure of work is often such that they are used simply as 'pairs of hands'. Project 2000 aims to make nursing more attractive as a career and to create a nursing workforce capable of adapting to the increasingly fast changing demands of the the health service and the profession. Thus, in addition to addressing long felt deficiencies in nursing education, it also offers the prospect of more efficient use of registered nurses. Project 2000 will:

Exhibit 4
THE ROLE OF THE NURSE (3)
Nurses are best placed to co-ordinate patient care and to represent patients

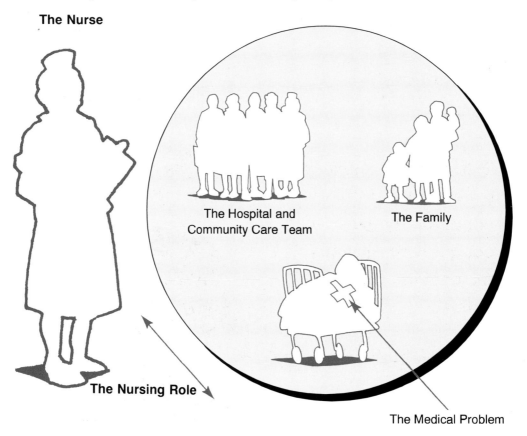

Source: Audit Commission

6

— **educate nurses alongside other students**, increasing their experience of the outside world and the academic content of their education;

— **make students supernumerary to ward establishments** for the first two years of their course;

— **replace a substantial portion of students' contribution** to the wards with a new breed of Health Care Support Worker;

— **phase out the second level of qualified nurse** by ending the training of enrolled nurses (ENs) and encouraging existing ENs to convert to registered (RGN) status.

10. On completion of their course, project 2000 nurses are likely to have a different outlook on nursing. And the role of the nurse may be changed more fundamentally by employment of more ward based support workers to take over responsibility for the ward environment.

WHAT CONSTITUTES 'GOOD' NURSING?

11. Despite ambiguity in the nurse's role and difficulty in measuring nursing outcomes, there is a fair consensus about what constitutes good nursing. Florence Nightingale was the first to recognise that nursing is about taking care of the *person who is ill*, rather than their medical problems, (Exhibit 5). Nowadays, the mechanism nurses use to translate the concept of individualised patient care into everyday practice is the problem solving approach to planning and delivering care known as **the nursing process**:

— on admission, the patient's needs are assessed by a nurse who will also try to find out how he feels about his condition and any preferences concerning his hospital stay or care.

— she uses the assessment to develop a plan of care tailored to the needs of that particular patient. Ideally, she discusses the plan with other professionals working with that patient.

Exhibit 5
PATIENT CENTRED CARE
Recognition that care should be dictated by the needs of each individual patient originated with
Florence Nightingale

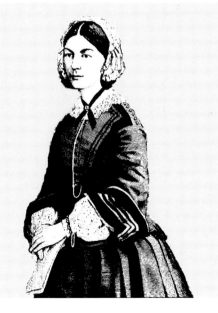

'It is better to know the patient in a certain condition than the condition from which the patient may suffer'

Florence Nightingale

— the patient is cared for in accordance with the plan, which is documented in enough detail for any nurse to look after the patient knowledgeably.

— the plan of care states specific care goals and review dates. If the care does not have the desired effect, or the patient's condition changes unexpectedly, the nurse reassesses his needs and amends the plan if necessary.

Nurses' attempts to make patient centred care a reality have stimulated many of the initiatives mentioned in this report.

12. The key distinguishing characteristic of good nursing is therefore that, as well as being founded on sound research-based practice, it puts the needs of the individual patient first. The Government's Patient's Charter (Ref. 5) recognises that the determination of these needs and the consistency with which they are met are most likely improve if each patient has a named nurse responsible for planning and overseeing his care from admission to discharge. If this standard is to be implemented meaningfully it will, in many hospitals, require significant changes in the way nursing staff work and are managed.

HOW THIS REPORT CAN HELP

13. This report seeks to show that there is considerable scope to enhance the quality of nursing within existing resource constraints and to bring current practice closer to the 'ideal' of good nursing described above. Action needs to be taken both by general managers and by ward sisters. This report focuses on what the higher levels of general and nursing management within provider units need to do. Two subsequent papers will be published, aimed at ward sisters and middle management. One suggests ways in which the change towards a named nurse for each patient could be implemented by ward sisters with the guidance and support of their immediate managers, largely within the resources already available to them. The other describes best practice in the use of nursing management systems and will be of prime interest to those responsible for choosing and implementing such systems.

14. This first report moves from discussion of outcomes, indicators of quality of care, through the processes of care delivery and the staffing needed to deliver that care, to underlying structures and the role of nursing management (Exhibit 6).

Section 1 starts from the patient's bedside, identifying systemic deficiencies in the care currently received by many patients and outlining ways in which that care might be improved.

Section 2 considers the numbers and skill-mix of nurses needed. It finds weaknesses in the use of nursing resources at ward level and describes the methods some hospitals have used to address them.

Section 3 looks at the management of nursing services in hospital and recommends ways of making it more effective.

Each section within these chapters first paints a picture of the ideal situation, then discusses problems which stand in the way of achieving this ideal, and finally sets out what general and nursing management must do to promote and monitor improvement. A summary of recommendations is included in the final chapter.

Exhibit 6
STRUCTURE OF THE REPORT
The report first discusses quality of care, then care processes, structures and finally management of the nursing service.

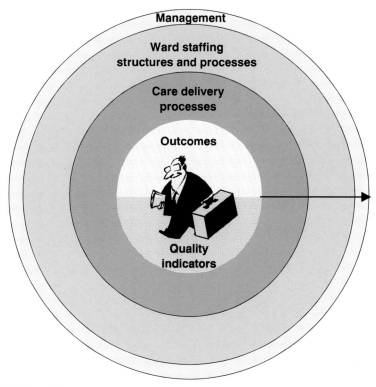

Source: Audit Commission

1. Delivering Better Patient Care

MEASURING QUALITY TO IMPROVE CARE

15. How good are current standards of nursing care? The question can not be answered definitively. In the absence of satisfactory outcome measures, proxy measures are needed. These include:

— patient perceptions,

— easily quantifiable indicators which may raise questions about quality of care,

— assessments of the way nursing care is delivered and of the ward environment.

16. All these aspects, not just clinical considerations, should inform priorities for quality improvement. Much of the detailed work on improving quality should be led by ward nurses themselves using quality *assurance* structures and procedures discussed below. But periodic quality *assessment* is also necessary if managers are to fulfil their duty of ensuring that basic standards of nursing care are not neglected. It helps managers to identify underlying reasons for problems common to a number of wards, some of which it may be outside the power of individual wards to correct. Such ideal arrangements are rarely found. Most hospitals do not systematically monitor patient opinion or the views of staff on the quality of care they are able to deliver. Most do not centrally collect and monitor those quality indicators that are available. And by no means all systematically audit the processes of nursing care.

Box A

Problems	Management Solutions
In the absence of satisfactory measures of nursing outcomes:	
(a) insufficient attention is paid to patient opinion and the views of ward staff on quality of care.	Better use of patient opinion surveys. Analysis of themes underlying comment and complaint.
(b) proxy measures are not being collected and used.	Indicators, e.g: incidence/change in size and severity of pressure sores, hospital acquired infections, drug errors, patient falls.
(c) not all hospitals conduct annual audits of the quality of the nursing process.	Use simple packages to monitor key trends and identify areas for fuller investigations.

PROBLEMS

(a) Insufficient Attention is paid to patient and staff opinion

17. To the majority of patients, nurses are still 'angels'. The number of gifts and donations from grateful patients bears testimony to their views. But a recent survey (reference 6) suggests underlying concern about some aspects of the nursing care in NHS hospitals. Of the survey respondents who had been in hospital in the previous 12 months, 29 per cent were dissatisfied with the amount of information they had received from nurses, and 18 per cent felt the nurses had been too busy to attend to their individual needs. Responses to questions on nursing care from the opinion survey 'What the Patient Thinks' similarly suggest that many patients would like more information from nurses and doctors about their treatment and that they would like more say in what is done to them, (Exhibit 7).

Exhibit 7
WHAT THE PATIENT THINKS:
Many patients would like more information...

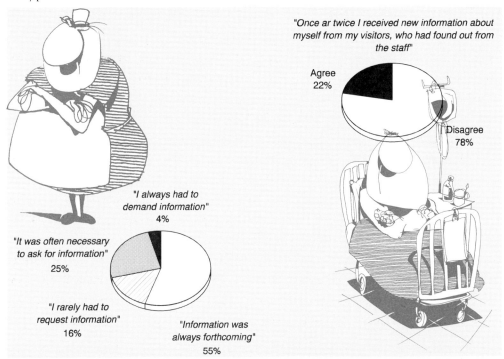

Source: Health Policy Advice Unit. Patients' opionions from general medical wards in 40 hospitals

18. Many hospitals provide patients with a form for comment on their stay. Outwardly, these questionnaires typically show that patients think standards of care are good. But the questions asked are often very general in nature with more emphasis on hotel services than on nursing care. Response rates are low and are sometimes depressed further by the arrangements made for the return of completed questionnaires. Patients frequently have low expectations and their opinions may be tempered by the sheer relief of being back at home or by the prospect of returning to the same hospital. Specific complaints about nursing are not common. When one does occur, most hospitals investigate the circumstances and provide a satisfactory response to the individual complainant. But far fewer systematically identify and remedy the underlying causes, which may for example be a lack of awareness of the importance of good communication.

12

(b) Insufficient use is made of quality indicators

19. Proxy measures or indicators of quality of care, with the possible exception of hospital acquired infections, are little used in NHS hospitals. Only one hospital studied routinely collated and analysed data on pressure sore incidence from all wards, although another was planning to introduce this as part of a 'basket' of indicators.

(c) Not all hospitals regularly audit care processes

20. Care audit packages are often used intermittently if at all, and sometimes only on a few wards. As a result, very few hospitals have systematic data going back in time to monitor trends in quality. Many methodologies are time-consuming and demanding for ward staff. A common source of frustration is that it can be a long time before the ward receives the results. Often the feedback is too general, and the tool too broad in its coverage or insufficiently selective, to allow nurses to pin-point the underlying problems in their practice.

MANAGEMENT SOLUTIONS

21. Some hospitals collect patient opinion in ways that *can* provide useful insights into what needs to be done to improve nursing care. Indicators are being refined and used to give early warning of trends and to trigger action. Ward audits are tailored to provide information useful to nurses and managers.

(a1) Ask the Patients

22. Patient opinion survey questions need to be specific rather than general and the sampling of the patient population statistically sound. Where response rates are poor, reasons should be analysed. Some hospitals are experimenting successfully with alternative methods of finding out what patients think about their treatment and care. One nurse manager interviewed conducts a structured interview with a sample of patients on her unit just before they are discharged. The ward sisters at a private hospital carry out exit interviews with *all* the patients, and an independent quality assurance department follows up a sample of patients at home. Some hospitals are trying to use the complaints system more positively, encouraging patient feedback and following up individual complaints to see if there are general as well as specific lessons to be learned.

(a2) Ask the nurses

23. Some hospitals ask the nurse in charge of each shift to rate care given on her ward during that period against a simple scale of quality and comment on contributory factors. This process, originally introduced to help managers assess the adequacy of ward staffing, also provides a continuous record of trends in quality of care as perceived by the nurses.

(b) Use indicators of care

24. There are a number of potentially valuable indicators of the quality of nursing care being delivered, for example:

— the incidence and rate of change in the size or severity of pressure sores,

— hospital-acquired infections,

— patient falls and other injuries to patients or staff,

— medication errors.

25. Indicators such as these are routinely collected and used in American hospitals and are scrutinised as part of the accreditation process. In Britain many nurses argue that they could reflect unfairly on wards since none convey an unambiguous message. A total absence of patient falls may for instance indicate an unduly restrictive regime rather than ideal care. But, if interpreted sensitively, indicators can be of value. Nurse managers in one hospital found, on investigating an increasing incidence of pressure sores, that this was due to deficiencies in care provided by local nursing homes before patients were admitted to hospital. Their matrons were alerted and guidance on modern techniques offered. Elsewhere high levels of drug errors were variously traced to faulty intravenous pumps and to difficulty in interpreting a doctor's handwriting. This enabled prompt remedial action to be taken.

26. There is enough evidence of the value of monitoring proxy indicators of the quality of care to justify their use as part of the nursing management system of any hospital.

(c) Audit care processes regularly.

27. 'Off-the-shelf' methods such as MONITOR and QUALPACS for measuring the quality of nursing care and the ward environment have their individual shortcomings, but they could be used much more widely and systematically. Some hospitals and health authorities have developed their own simpler quality assessment packages which require less staff resources and so can be used more frequently. And at some hospitals, the annual ward audits carried out by schools of nursing have been developed explicitly to provide information that is useful to managers of the service as well as for educational purposes. The inspections are planned and carried out jointly by the school and the hospital. If audits and inspections are to be effective, results should be fed back to ward staff promptly. They may need help interpreting the results and using them to change their practice. An action plan should be agreed and followed up by managers.

QUALITY ASSURANCE

28. There should be a shared commitment throughout the hospital to continuous quality improvement. Ideally nurses would participate with doctors and other professions in auditing how patients are treated in hospital and in researching the outcomes of different modes of care. Their findings would then be reflected in research based procedural guidance and standards. Other ward-specific nursing standards would be developed, within the context of an agreed meaningful ward philosophy, to address care issues of particular relevance or concern to patients and staff on that ward. These standards would include measurable quality or outcome objectives for key aspects of nursing care and details of the resources and procedures needed to meet them. Regular monitoring of standards would act as a spring-board for further improvement.

29. Nursing, as a profession, places great emphasis on quality of care. But efforts to improve care processes are not everywhere conducted within a framework set by senior managers. They are seldom planned systematically or informed by the concerns of patients. Nor are the outcomes of quality initiatives systematically monitored and evaluated.

Box B

	Problems	Management Solutions
(d)	Quality Assurance approaches such as standard setting can be: – Patchy – Misdirected and irrelevant to actual problems.	Adopt an approach similar to DYSSSY:- management provides a structure and support for QA, but standards are owned by ward staff and specific to problems of ward.
(e)	There is a lack of multi-disciplinary clinical audit.	Promote nursing involvement in clinical audit. Expand role of NDUs in developing and publicising good practice.

PROBLEMS

(d) Patchy and misdirected effort on standard setting

30. Nurses in some hospitals put a lot of effort into writing ward philosophies and nursing standards. But there are marked differences in the way this is done:

— At some hospitals, standards are formulated by senior nurses as an extension of procedural regulations with little or no consultation with ward nurses. Many ward staff show little awareness of these standards;

— Elsewhere each ward is instructed by management to produce a standard on a specified topic. These are collated and disseminated to all wards, regardless of relevance to the type of patients treated or to nurses' perceptions of priorities for quality improvement. Typically little guidance is provided on writing or monitoring standards;

— In some places standard writing is delegated to enthusiasts. Where formal structures are lacking, there is considerable duplication of effort. Support from senior nurses may be limited. Nurses may be unable to obtain sufficient resources to implement the standards or they may address areas that should properly be actioned by management.

31. Thus in some hospitals standard writing has little effect on care received by patients. Many existing standards do not have quantified targets and only one of the hospitals in the study had effective arrangements for monitoring compliance. And, because of lack of guidance, ward philosophies written at the behest of management are often empty generalised statements languishing in a drawer. In such cases they are of little lasting value and do not serve as a guiding framework for ward-based standards.

(e) Lack of multidisciplinary clinical audit

32. At a few hospitals doctors invite nurses into *medical audit* sessions, but at all except one in the Audit Commission sample, *nursing care audit* is proceeding separately. For the time being, this has the advantage that nurses are able to gain in confidence and issues of special interest to them are high on the agenda, but in the longer term it is not in the patient's interest for each professional group to develop its own set of standards independently of the rest.

MANAGEMENT SOLUTIONS

(d) Establishing a framework for nursing standards

33. The Royal College of Nursing's Dynamic Standard Setting System (DySSSy) is one example of an approach which provides a framework set and controlled by hospital management within which groups of nurses write and evaluate ward based standards. It gives guidance on how to measure the resources and actions that will be needed to achieve the standard and, where possible, how to measure the effect on outcomes. Features of DySSSy are :-

— 'Ownership' of the resulting standards by nurses which improves understanding of their purpose and motivation to take appropriate action.

— Participation and involvement of all practitioners working in the area where the standard applies, leading eventually to multi-disciplinary standards for patient care.

— Recognition of the need to provide resources and time to facilitate the standard setting process.

— Focus on demonstrable improvement to patient care in areas of current concern to all nurses on the ward or where problems have been identified by clinicians or management.

— Achievability in the face of likely resource constraints. A requirement that each standard be signed off by the Director of Nursing Services or a senior manager ensures influential backing for its implementation.

34. A number of hospitals are successfully using this approach to standard setting to improve care. One ward caring for elderly patients used DySSSy to develop a standard which on implementation cut the incidence of pressure sores from 26 to 7 per cent. This has clear value. Serious pressure sores cause considerable pain, lengthen hospital stays and are expensive to treat:- a study in one district estimated the cost at more than £25,000 per patient (Ref. 7).

35. A similar approach has been used for some years in a leading American hospital. All nurses on each 'floor' (the equivalent of a UK ward), participate in monthly meetings to set and revise standards. Each floor sends a representative to a hospital-wide co-ordinating committee which shares information on standards produced and agrees follow up. All standards must include a specification of how they will be evaluated. But once initial improvement targets have been achieved, monitoring is suspended for an agreed period or until there is again cause for concern so as not to waste effort on expensive data collection. Standard setting work moves on to new areas of interest.

(e1) Nursing involvement in clinical audit

36. Managers will need to take a lead if truly *multi-disciplinary* clinical audit is to be established. A first step would be to facilitate identification of topics of common concern to doctors and nurses and exchange of views or information on factors relevant to both medical and nursing audit. A constructive parallel development is the formation of *quality circles* and other interdisciplinary staff groups at a number of hospitals to discuss problems or concerns about patient care and to spread ideas on good practice.

(e2) Promoting research into nursing practice
– the contribution of nursing development units

37. As already noted, there has been little research into the effectiveness of nursing practice, or the relationship between resources and quality of care. Some American hospitals are attempting to fill this gap by giving each employee a stake in improving patient care. Some have introduced clinical ladders. To progress their career, nurses must give a presentation on their

contribution to an aspect of care. All nurses are committed to researching the outcome of their work to the best of their ability. They are given facilities and academic support to enable this and their achievements are recognised by management.

38. The *nursing development units* (NDUs) that have been set up by a number of units, usually with special funds from the district or with the help of the Kings Fund, offer the potential for replicating this success in Britain. One, for example, is evaluating benefits for patients of different forms of primary nursing (see below), concentrating initially on measuring improvement in communication between nurses and patients. NDUs are ordinary wards or clinics that are committed to developing nursing practice, measuring the outcomes and spreading good ideas. The additional funding typically pays for support to enable the ward sister to spend time publicising the work of the unit and for a supernumerary research nurse. £3.2 millions have recently been made available by the Department of Health to expand these schemes. To be effective agents of change, NDUs need the support and commitment of management. The need for a stable ward environment within which ongoing research can be evaluated should be taken into consideration if ward closures or amalgamations are necessary. Nurse managers should also adopt a more positive stance towards spreading innovative practice from NDUs to other wards in their own hospitals and districts.

MAKING CARE MORE PATIENT CENTRED

39. Patients prefer to be cared for as individuals, and not as either bodies in bed or medical diagnoses ('the CVA in the side room'). A large scale survey (Ref. 8) based on 'What the Patient Thinks' shows that patients rate wards providing more patient centred care higher than others dominated by routines.

40. Such evidence as is available from small scale studies in surgery and oncology suggests that the extent to which care is patient centred is also a key determinant of quality. The recent report by the College of Anaesthetists and Royal College of Surgeons on the management of post-operative pain (Ref. 9) for example underlines the importance of the nurses' role, and the need for care to be tailored much more carefully to the individual patient to achieve effective pain control and speed the patient's recovery. With other research studies (Ref. 10), it confirms the importance of patients' active participation in treatment, and the reduction in their levels of anxiety that occurs when they are given information about their condition and treatment.

41. The introduction of the Nursing Process throughout Britain in the 1980s should have ensured that care was tailored better to the needs of the individual. But this has not happened everywhere. Some wards continue to be run by routines and almost everywhere care planning and documentation remains poor. Scant account is usually taken of patients' preferences as to when and how care is given.

Box C

	Problems	Management solutions
(f)	Ward run by routines – all patients get similar care (e.g. termperatures, timing of medication) regardless of clinical need.	More information for nurse managers on how wards are run. More professional development. Improve liaison with doctors.
(g)	Poor planning and documentation of care needs. (Continuity of responsibility for care of individuals given low priority).	Show good planning matters (by giving it priority and time). Periodic audit of care plans. Continuous responsibility for care of each individual patient allocated to a qualified nurse who knows that patient.

FACTORS INHIBITING PATIENT CENTRED CARE

(f) Unnecessary Ward Routines

42. Thirty years ago an official report recommended that the practice of waking patients between 5 and 6 a.m. should end (Ref. 11). The rationale for waking *every* patient on the ward early, rather than only those whose clinical treatment demands it, was that night staff needed to complete their allotted tasks before going off-duty. A majority of patients would prefer not to be woken so early, and yet it is still common practice on many wards, (Exhibit 8). On some wards where early waking is routine, the morning handover does not take place until *after* care has been given to patients for some time by the oncoming early shift, increasing the risk that inappropriate or non-individualised care will be given. Other examples of routines that may be imposed on patients unthinkingly or for the convenience of staff include getting all patients washed and their beds tidied first thing in the morning before the doctor's rounds and giving pain killing drugs at set times regardless of need. And on a few wards studied, visiting times are still limited to one

Exhibit 8
UNNECESSARY ROUTINES
A majority of patients feel that they have to fit in with set routines . . .   . . . but would prefer not to be woken so early.

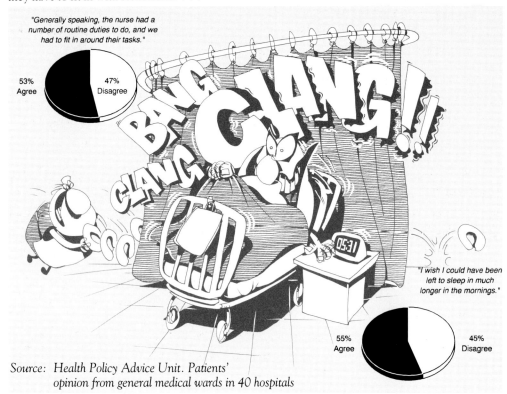

Source: *Health Policy Advice Unit. Patients'*
opinion from general medical wards in 40 hospitals

hour per evening, whereas patients with very similar conditions on other wards welcome open visiting.

(g) Poor Care Planning and Documentation

43. Despite the investment by many hospitals over a number of years in training, standards of care planning and record keeping are generally poor. On some wards, care plans are so incomplete that a nurse new to the ward would not find in them sufficient information to give acceptable care to her patients. Poor quality care planning and record keeping does not *necessarily* indicate poor quality patient care. But unless verbal communication between nurses on the ward is outstanding, it does mean that care can not be tailored specifically to the patient. For this *all* the nurses involved with the patient need access to information about his needs, preferences, what he has or has not been told, and the latest developments in his treatment. There are a number of reasons why care plans are completed only perfunctorily for most patients and convey very little individual detail:-

44. **Care planning is given insufficient priority**: Care planning is often seen mainly as a training exercise for students. Plans are written up just before nurses go off-duty, or even at home (in which case they will not be available to nurses on the in-coming shift). Many nurses see 'writing up the notes' as a task that takes them away from the patient's bedside. And some consultants' negative attitude towards nurses 'spending too much time filling in forms' reinforces such views. Emphasis may be placed on finding ways of producing care plans more quickly, for instance by inappropriate extension of the use of standardised care plans for patients undergoing certain procedures, rather than on improving the value of their content.

45. **The assessment may be carried out by the wrong person**: Assessment should only be undertaken by a trained nurse or by a student under supervision. At one hospital, nurses were not aware of this requirement. At others, when the ward was short-staffed, an experienced auxiliary completed patients' assessments. In a few cases this could put patients at risk. It may also lead to provision of *too much* of the *wrong sort* of nursing care. An elderly patient might for instance wrongly be assumed to be incontinent or unable to walk without assistance.

46. **Care may be planned by a nurse who does not know the patient**: Care plans are not always written by a nurse who is directly involved in caring for the patient or who is accountable for that care. Sometimes care is planned by night staff during unoccupied time. Most of these nurses would not have had a chance to observe or talk to the patient during his waking hours.

47. **The design of patient documentation could be better adapted to its use:** Despite the lack of individualisation, nursing documentation is often lengthy. Information about the patient may be divided between the nursing notes (or 'Kardex'), the care plan, sister's diary and the notes nurses make for themselves at handover. It can be difficult to locate details in a hurry. There is also considerable duplication between all these sources and case notes made by other professionals.

MANAGEMENT SOLUTIONS

48. Patient centred care can not be imposed by managers. Ward nurses must be convinced of the necessity for change and take the lead in developing their practice. With a few exceptions,

developments have been led by enthusiasts on one or two wards in some hospitals and have then percolated outwards. The management role is one of urging, facilitation, monitoring and audit.

(f) Getting rid of unnecessary routines

49. Research suggests that nurses rely so much on routines partly because of the lack of stability in the staffing of wards from shift to shift, (Ref. 12). It can be argued that in some hospitals and wards it is exacerbated by a lack of focused professional development and exposure to alternative ways of working. Both of these topics are discussed in Chapter 2. But before the problem can be addressed, many nurse managers will need more information on how their wards are run.

(g) Recognising the importance of care planning

50. Tailoring care to the specific needs of the individual patient takes time. Nurses on the best general medical wards in the Audit Commission study spend an average of 40 minutes per patient per day – 20 percent of their time – planning, evaluating and documenting care. But they say that this investment in individually planned care can lead to a net *saving* of nursing time by eliminating unnecessary and time-consuming routines (such as regular recording of temperatures, blood pressure and bowel movements) that for certain patients serve no clinical purpose. Research to date into the extent and effects of 'over-' and 'under-nursing' is comparatively sparse and largely confined to wards caring for the elderly. But it is claimed that better planning is also likely to facilitate rehabilitation and reduce the risk of complications which may delay discharge or lead to readmission. Where the plan is agreed with the other professionals involved in caring for the patient it is often possible to improve the quality of the patient's stay. In many cases, for instance, it is not necessary to wake patients at 6 a.m. for medication and,between them, doctors and nurses can devise more patient centred regimes.

51. Managers can facilitate the improved liaison between nurses and doctors that is necessary for a common appreciation of the value of good care planning based on discussion of how care can best be delivered to individual patients. Managers also need to show that *they* recognise it as a priority and provide nurses with time to do it well. This should be reinforced by periodic audit of care plans by senior nurses. A number of hospitals are introducing computerised care planning systems to speed up the clerical element of the process. The advantages, (consistency and legibility) and disadvantages (less individualisation in some instances) of computerisation are discussed in the companion paper on the use of nursing management systems.

ARE THESE SOLUTIONS SUFFICIENT?

52. It has been argued that there is more incentive for a nurse to plan and document care well if she is responsible for the care given to a patient throughout his hospital stay and has the satisfaction of seeing the results of her own, and her colleagues', work with that patient. If this is so, improving the continuity of care must be a key factor in making care more patient centred.

IMPROVING CONTINUITY OF CARE

53. The 'Patient's Charter' states:

'the charter standard is that you should have a named, qualified nurse, midwife or health visitor who will be responsible for your nursing or midwifery care', (Ref. 5)

Previewing this, the Prime Minister said that a patient could expect the named nurse to be responsible for his care *'from start to finish'*. This has been interpreted by many nurses as a commitment to introduce *primary nursing* throughout the NHS. Each 'primary nurse' has 24 hour responsibility and authority over all aspects of the nursing care of a small group of patients throughout their stay. She is typically responsible for between six and eight patients of average dependency at a time on a general medical ward. Since she can be on duty for only part of the day, she is assisted in *delivering* care by three or four named associate nurses or support workers.

HOW IS CARE ORGANISED AT PRESENT?

54. Primary nursing is a continuation of a trend in the way nursing care is organised on the wards. This has evolved over recent years from the allocation of *tasks* to nurses, one dressing all the patients whilst another attended to their skin care, to allocation of responsibility for the *complete care of a group of patients*. But the way nursing care is organised at present can be very different from one ward to another, even within the same hospital. On 40 per cent of the wards studied, nurses may be allocated *different* patients from shift to shift. On 45 per cent, a team of nurses takes responsibility for specific areas of the ward. Continuity of care on some of these wards is excellent. But elsewhere if, as often happens, patients change beds they may also change teams. Some teams 'swap ends' weekly or more frequently 'to even up the workload' or 'because the nurses don't find working all the time with the heavy patients stimulating'. Just 6 out of the 39 wards studied (15%) have already adopted primary nursing (Exhibit 9, overleaf).

55. There is no conclusive research evidence on the effectiveness of primary nursing in improving clinical outcomes in ways that can be quantified. This is so even in those American Hospitals where it has been the norm for some years. However patients like it. And there is a ground-swell of professional opinion in its favour. It offers the best, but not the only way of promoting continuity of care for each patient. This, it is argued, reduces the risk of accidental omission or error. It improves communication between patients and health professionals. It reduces avoidable delays in making decisions about changes needed to patient care. And it helps to ensure that appropriate arrangements are made for patients' discharges. What is more, it could improve efficiency because, if care is delivered consistently according to a plan designed specifically for each patient, unnecessary routines are eliminated.

WHY HAS CHANGE BECOME NECESSARY?

56. In the past the ward sister provided continuity on the ward because she knew, or seemed to know, everything about every patient. On most wards, it is no longer possible for ward sisters to fulfil this function. The clinical condition of many patients changes too rapidly, and there are too many people – patients passing through the ward and the health professionals involved with them – for one person to be able to keep in touch with what is happening at all times. These, together with the reductions in the length of nurses' working week, have made complete familiarity with everyone and everything on the ward impossible. Greater delegation of responsibility for patient care to staff nurses is becoming inevitable. Under primary nursing, the ward sister may take a small primary nurse caseload herself, or may fill in as an associate nurse. But her main role becomes one of clinical consultant to the other nurses, teacher, facilitator and staff manager.

Exhibit 9
ORGANISATION OF CARE
The organisation of care can be very different from one ward to another, even within the same hospital

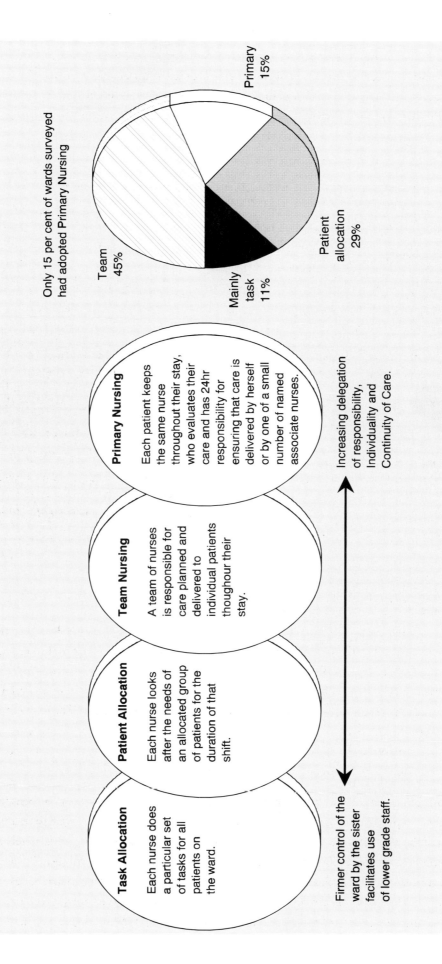

Only 15 per cent of wards surveyed had adopted Primary Nursing

Primary 15%

Patient allocation 29%

Mainly task 11%

Team 45%

Task Allocation

Each nurse does a particular set of tasks for all patients on the ward.

Patient Allocation

Each nurse looks after the needs of an allocated group of patients for the duration of that shift.

Team Nursing

A team of nurses is responsible for care planned and delivered to individual patients thoughour their stay.

Primary Nursing

Each patient keeps the same nurse throughout their stay, who evaluates their care and has 24hr responsibility for ensuring that care is delivered by herself or by one of a small number of named associate nurses.

Firmer control of the ward by the sister facilitates use of lower grade staff.

Increasing delegation of responsibility, Individuality and Continuity of Care.

Source: Audit Commission

22

57. The spread of primary nursing is therefore welcome. But there will be problems in implementing it successfully. Those likely to stem from the way certain wards are staffed at present are discussed in Chapter 2. Other obstacles are examined first. Unless the change is carefully managed and monitored, the 'named nurse' will not be able to exercise her responsibility effectively and old deficiencies in care could be perpetuated under a new name.

Box D

	Problems	Management solutions
(h)	Terminology can be misleading. Not all wards claiming to operate primary nursing can guarantee that patients are looked after by a nurse who knows them when the primary nurse is off-duty.	Managers will need more information about organisation of care. Better rostering and more stable ward staffing. Clarify responsibility for staffing ward at night. Avoid ward transfers if possible.
	Transfer of patients between wards negates benefits of primary nursing.	
(i)	Not all nurses are ready to take on the responsibility of becoming a primary nurse.	Introduce good 'team nursing' first. Improve professional development.
(j)	Communication between nurses and with doctors and patients could be better.	Management support for initiatives taken by nurses to cut out intermediaries when communicating with doctors and patients.
(k)	Discharge planning is ofter too little and too late, with no follow-up.	Discharge policy supported by training, monitoring, feedback, including need to assess discharge requirements from admission.
	Preparation for discharge is patchy.	Provide resources, support for improved patient information.

PROBLEMS IN MAKING CONTINUITY OF CARE A REALITY
(h) Terminology of care organisation can be misleading

58. Terms such as patient allocation, team nursing and primary nursing by which nurses commonly categorise the different approaches to organising care can cause confusion because they are not used consistently. In practice, the boundaries between them are blurred. Organisation of care can also vary between shifts. For instance, although task allocation has virtually disappeared as a *planned* method of organising care, the proportion of work still actually undertaken on this basis increases considerably outside the 'early' shift. Thus some wards operating primary nursing still have very task oriented delivery of care at nights and during periods when wards are short staffed or are heavily reliant on temporary staff or students.

59. It is important to patients that they know who is looking after them on each shift as well as who is responsible for planning their care. Without this knowledge, how can patients know which of the nurses to talk to about what is happening? Who is the right person to tell when their symptoms change? Who can answer their questions? Certain patients may benefit clinically from continuity of relationships with a small group of nurses because the trust that develops makes it easier for the nurses to identify and treat problems that inhibit the patient's recovery. But patients on the majority of wards studied did *not* know which nurse or group of nurses was

responsible for looking after them. Transfer of patients between wards for other than clinical reasons (noted in the Audit Commission report on the use of medical beds, (Ref. 13), and prevalent in most hospitals studied) also destroys continuity of care and complicates discharge planning.

(i) Are nurses ready for the additional responsibility?

60. Not all nurses are ready for the responsibility of becoming a primary nurse. For many it will be a big culture change. Only some of the care delivered by nurses is prescribed by a doctor. The rest is up to them. Under the UKCC Code of Conduct, each qualified nurse is clearly professionally accountable for her own *actions*. But at present on many wards there is a lack of clear responsibility for making *decisions* affecting the care given to a patient. Staff nurses *and* the ward sister are accountable, but neither feels fully responsible. The nurse caring for the patient may be required to refer significant decisions to the nurse in charge who is less likely to know the full picture. And at the end of the shift responsibility is passed to another set of staff. Many wards have initially experienced high staff turnover when they introduced primary nursing, with nurses transferring to areas where work was organised on more familiar lines, (Ref. 14). But those wards usually had a queue of applicants who wanted the challenge of working in a pioneering environment. This will not be so when all wards are making the change.

(j) Communication must be improved

61. **Communication with patients and relatives:** A hospital stay can be a lonely, bewildering, and frightening, as well as a boring experience for many people. One patient, describing her experience for the *Nursing Times* wrote (Ref. 15):

> 'If a nurse had sat down on my bed, touched or held my hand and asked: 'What are you thinking?' or 'How are you really feeling?', I would have been able to say that I felt trapped in a nightmare, that my life seemed ruined and that death appeared a viable option. By expressing these emotions, I might have felt less isolated, less stigmatised and a lot better.'

62. Good communication with patients contributes to more effective care, but nurses are sometimes inhibited in the information they are able to give by individual consultants' policies. On wards with more than one consultant it is not unusual for nurses to find that they are allowed by one to give patients information on request, but not by another.

63. **Communication between nurses:** Given the amount of time it takes to plan patients' care properly, it is important not to lose the potential benefit through poor verbal and written communication. Time available for handover between shifts is not always used to best effect. On many wards handover is still conducted between the *nurse in charge* of the previous shift and *all* the nurses on the in-coming shift. The nurse in charge does not always have first hand knowledge of the patients and although all the nurses need a small amount of key information about all the patients (e.g. the list of who is not for 'active treatment' and contagion status) they do not all need every patient's details. Much better use could be made of written records at handover and throughout the shift.

64. **Communication with doctors:** Even where responsibility for the care of specific patients has been devolved, it is still common for all calls to medical staff to go through the nurse in charge of the ward and for her to accompany consultants on their ward rounds.

(k) Poor Discharge Planning[*]

65. For many patients, the need for nursing care does not end on discharge from hospital. But communication between ward and community nurses is frequently at second-hand through a liaison nurse. Ward nurses usually bear the main responsibility for initiating and co-ordinating discharge planning, calling on other professions and support staff to make the practical arrangements. Although many hospitals have discharge policies and procedures, staff often either do not know about them or do not find them helpful. The practical administration of discharge remains poor and does not appear to have improved since the Department of Health published guidance in 1989 (Ref. 16). Assessment of the need for discharge planning is patchy, too late, and poorly documented. Many care plans have a discharge section but it is common for it to be left blank. In consequence discharge may be delayed, services inappropriate and avoidable readmissions may result.

66. **Preparation for Discharge** The amount of health education and information about support and services in the community that is available to patients in hospital varies considerably between similar wards. It sometimes varies between different consultants' patients on the same ward.

MANAGEMENT SOLUTIONS – IMPROVING CONTINUITY OF CARE
(h) Concentrate on the principles of continuity

67. Those monitoring implementation of primary nursing should concentrate on the extent to which the principles of continuity are observed. Have channels of communication – with patients and relatives, between nurses, and with other clinicians – been simplified by cutting out intermediaries? Are responsibilities for making decisions about patient care clear? Does one nominated nurse take the lead for each patient, changes in her absence being made only in emergencies? How many different nurses and auxiliaries on average are involved in physically caring for each patient during his stay? The key to better physical continuity of care on many wards is, as discussed in Chapter 2, better rostering of stable ward teams coupled with clarification of responsibility for how wards are staffed at night.

68. **Avoid ward transfers:** Ward transfers for other than medical reasons are not conducive to continuity of care. The Audit Commission report on use of medical beds recommends ways in which managers can reduce the frequency of transfers. If pressure of space makes a transfer essential, there must be an effective handover of responsibility for nursing care. In one hospital studied a standard has been introduced to ensure that only clinically and emotionally suitable patients are considered for transfer and that planned care is continued subsequently. The onus is put on the primary nurse from the transferring ward to discuss care needs with nurses on the receiving ward and to check up on the patient following the transfer. Other units have devised documentation to accompany the patient whenever he leaves the ward.

(i) Don't rush the change to primary nursing

69. The experience of pioneering wards shows that gradual evolution is necessary. Managers should not try to impose primary nursing without taking all the ward nurses and

---

[*]   *(Discharge planning arrangements are also discussed in forthcoming Audit Commission reports on the use of medical beds in acute hospitals and services in the community).*

auxiliaries with them. They should ensure that professional development is stepped up first so that all nurses appreciate the possibilities of change. It may be better for some wards to change first to one of the better types of team nursing, where patient-nurse allocation lasts the length of the patient's stay and the composition of the teams is comparatively stable.

(j) Better communication

70. **With patients**: Managers should ensure that nurses are trained to give information clearly and sensitively. They should try to ensure that nurses and doctors working on the same wards agree together an approach to information that is based on patients' needs and interests. They should feed back patient comment on the clarity and adequacy of information received.

71. **Between nurses**: Nurse managers can help to promote more efficient handovers. On the more progressive wards studied there is a very short office handover limited to key factual information about patients. The main handover is conducted in small groups between those nurses directly involved in caring for each patient, often at the patient's bedside. This gives more chance for questions, saves time and can, if done well, provide an opportunity for the patient to discuss his treatment and care with the nurses. Nurses at an American hospital visited are timing and analysing everything that happens during handover with the aim of making it more relevant to the patient. Some wards have found that tape-recorded commentaries are an efficient way of giving staff, particularly those who start part way through a shift, additional information about patients.

72. **With doctors**: In most instances, communication between nurses and doctors (and other professionals) is better, in the sense that it is more detailed, more up-to-date and more grounded in personal knowledge of the patient, when it involves the nurse caring for the patient. Management support may help to overcome initial resistance from doctors. Managers and ward sisters must make sure that other health professionals understand the reasons for change and that the objective of improved communication is achieved.

(k) Improved Discharge Planning

73. Each patient's needs for special discharge arrangements should be assessed soon after admission. Where there is a named nurse responsible for a patient's care, she should be invited to any subsequent multidisciplinary team meetings to discuss discharge. This practice is increasingly widespread, especially on care of the elderly wards. At two study sites, community nurses regularly visit the wards to discuss impending discharges. Nurses on some wards have taken the lead in providing patients with relevant pamphlets on preserving their health and coping with their conditions after discharge. They also provide directories of services and support groups that patients can contact. These are to be welcomed in principle. But research on their effectiveness and potential for reducing readmission rates would be valuable.

2. Staffing the Wards

74. It is axiomatic that, if care is to become more patient centred, ward staffing must reflect patients' needs. Many nurses would argue that to do so properly requires additional staff. Some also argue that primary nursing, if properly managed, needs a higher ratio of qualified staff to patients.

75. The overall level of staffing in NHS hospitals must be a matter for management decision within funds made available by government. But where there are pressures for additional resources, it is vital that existing staff are deployed in the most effective way. That means ensuring that ward establishments, skill mix and the availability of support staff are as closely aligned as they can be with workload. This chapter addresses ways in which that alignment can be promoted through regular reviews. It then goes on to discuss recruitment and retention and the development of clinical skills that would be needed to effect improvements in the standard of care. Finally it considers the day to day staffing of wards and the way in which nurses can be most effectively deployed to maximise the continuity of good quality care.

Box E
EMPLOYING THE 'RIGHT' NUMBERS AND MIX OF STAFF

Problems	Management solutions
Not Consensus on how many nurses or what skill mix are needed:	Put in place structures to evaluate change.
(a) Data is poor and there is no consistent approach to setting ward establishment.	Zero based, collaborative review of numbers & skill mix reflecting agreed workload for the ward.
The wide variation in staff numbers and between similar wards is not easily explained. It is not straightforward to effect change.	Facilitate activity analysis first and review resulting action plans. Workload assessment can inform periodic review of staffing if other uses are also encouraged.
(b) Non-nursing duties are common.	Facilitate negotiated change to skill-mix within agreed budgets to meeet patient need. Cost non-nursing duties when reviewing support services.
(c) Confusion about effects of Project 2000 implementation.	Improve co-ordination of planning and communication.

PROBLEMS IN DETERMINING HOW MANY NURSES ARE NEEDED?
LACK OF RESEARCH LINKING STAFFING TO OUTCOMES

76. There can be no clear answer to the question 'how many nurses are needed?'. It has been claimed that:

'nursing establishments are determined more by rhetoric, historical accident and well intentioned guesses than by scientific evaluation of the needs of the individual patient', (Ref. 17).

This is true of many professions in the NHS. But there is certainly a lack of conclusive evidence on the effect of variations in ward staffing on care *outcomes*.

(a1) National data does not permit meaningful comparisons

77. No data is routinely collected nationally which permits broad comparison of the staffing of wards of similar size and specialty. Health service indicators show large variations between districts, both in the average *numbers* of qualified nurses per patient day and in the *proportions* of qualified staff employed in acute wards, but can be misleading (Exhibit 10). Some of this variation may be due to differences in the case-mix of patients treated by each district (for instance the presence or otherwise of regional specialties and academic departments may call for higher levels of technical skill amongst nurses) and some to the availability of student nurses. Some is explained by defects in the data.

Exhibit 10
ACUTE WARD STAFFING
National statistics suggest large variations between Health Authorities in the average number of Qualified Nurses per Patient Day in Acute Wards

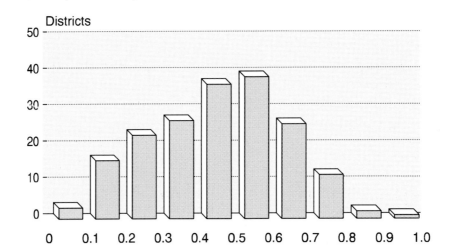

There is correspondingly wide variation in the Proportion of Nurses in Acute Wards who are Qualified

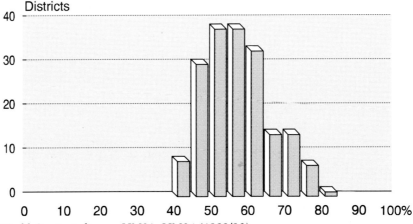

Source: Health Service indicators HN21, HN24 (1989/90)

Note: Excludes Special Health Authorities, Districts with less than 50 nurses or claiming impossibly high activity.

28

(a2) Wide variation in ward establishments is not easily explained

78. To gain a better impression of the true extent of variation in ward staffing, data on establishments and staff in post, together with average allocations of students and pool nurses, were collected from the 39 general medical and surgical wards studied by the Audit Commission. Figures were adjusted to compensate for differences in the way wards were staffed at night. The staffing of these wards is clearly related to the average number of patients. This relationship is improved if one half of the average number of learners actually present on each ward (generally a roughly equal number of first and third year students) during the six months preceding the study is added to the adjusted 24 hour ward establishment. (A number of workload assessment systems provide a precedent for counting learners' contribution to patient care as a proportion of that made by a permanent member of the ward team).

79. Although staffing is related to patient numbers, a core of about a dozen staff appears to be necessary simply to administer the ward and provide minimum safe cover over a 24 hour period throughout the year (Exhibit 11). *Much of the variation in nurse-patient ratios shown by the Health Service Indicators therefore simply reflects differences in ward sizes.* On average, an increased establishment of one additional nurse is provided for every three patients present. But there is still variation of over 20 per cent in the staffing of wards of similar size and occupancy. This is not explained by the throughput of patients, their age, sex, the mix of cases, patients' lengths of stay or the layout of the ward. The lack of a commonly accepted measure of patient dependency or nursing workload prevents more detailed analysis.

Exhibit 11
GENERAL MEDICAL/SURGICAL WARD STAFFING
Staffing is related to numbers of patients but a core of about a dozen is required to administer the ward and provide minimum safe cover

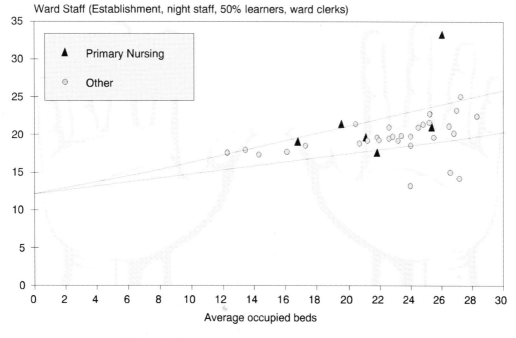

Ward Staff (Establishment, night staff, 50% learners, ward clerks)

Source: Audit Commission Site Visits

Note: 1) *High outiler was until recently two separate wards*
       2) *Low outilers, all in one hospital, also use pool nurses*

80. **Does primary nursing require more staff?** It is often assumed that additional staff are required to introduce primary nursing. But three of the six wards studied who currently practise primary nursing had below average staffing levels in relation to their size and occupancy. And, despite a higher grade mix, not all of them had markedly above average staffing costs (Exhibit 12). This sample is too small for generalised conclusions to be drawn. The local audits based on this study will provide data on staffing, activity and organisation of care from about a thousand wards across the country. This may help to determine the relative costs of primary nursing.

Exhibit 12
GENERAL MEDICAL/SURGICAL WARD STAFF COSTS
COMPARED TO AVERAGE OCCUPIED BEDS
Not all primary nursing wards have above average staff costs

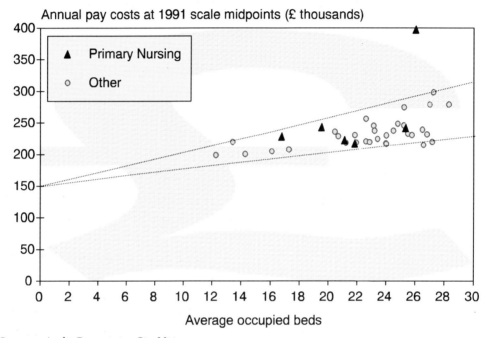

Source: Audit Commission Site Visits

Note: Includes basic pay costs (at scale midpoints) of ward nursing staff, night staff, learners and ward clerks. High outlier was until recently two separate wards

81. **Wide variation in current skill mix** National trends have been towards a more skilled general nursing workforce in acute hospitals. The overall percentage of qualified nursing staff rose from 53.5 to 57.2 between 1985 and 1989. But locally there is significant variation. On general medical wards included in the study it varied between 38 and 72 per cent, (Exhibit 13). On one ward almost half of the normal staffing was provided by learners whilst others had no pre-registration students. The proportion of auxiliaries and other untrained staff on these wards ranged from 5 to 22 per cent. These findings confirm the extent of variation reported by previous studies (Ref. 18 and 19).

82. Such comparative data on the staffing of outwardly similar wards across the country can provoke questions. But local factors and differences in the quality of care provided on wards with differing levels and mix of staffing and availability of support services must be taken into consideration when reviewing ward staffing before useful conclusions can be drawn about potential efficiency improvements.

Exhibit 13
SKILL MIX ON THREE GENERAL MEDICAL WARDS
There is significant variation of skill-mix

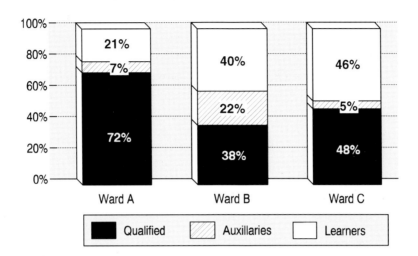

Source: *Audit Commission Site Visits*
        (Funded Establishments – 3 Different Hospitals)

(a3) The difficulty of changing ward establishments

83. It is generally accepted that ward establishments should be regularly reviewed. But reviews are complex and the results are often difficult to implement. So in practice they happen infrequently. Instead, ward staffing is changed incrementally as different nurse managers, ward sisters and consultants bring their influence to bear or as workload changes. The current grade mix of staff on wards is frequently determined more by the way duties were performed at the time clinical grading was introduced than by the needs of patients.

84. Many hospitals have placed too great an emphasis on the value of workload systems for reviewing establishments and not enough on other potential uses. One hospital, for example, has collected workload data which appears to show a consistent and significant shortfall in numbers of staff daily for two years, without changing staffing levels. Not surprisingly, ward staff, who make no use of the data themselves, are cynical about the value of the system and data entry has become intermittent and inaccurate. Although workload data can be a valuable input to establishment review, the cost-justification of compiling daily or shift-by-shift dependency or task data over a number of years *solely* for this purpose must be questionable. It is important also to recognise its limitations. The different workload assessment methodologies in use can suggest considerably different staffing requirements. Some require local calibration. This is bound to reflect current working practices as well as the individual features of each ward and its patients. Thus although the consistency with which each ward within a hospital is staffed in relation to patient needs may be improved, comparison of staffing levels with those of other hospitals is likely to remain problematic.

(b) Inappropriate duties

85. On the majority of wards studied, qualified nurses confirmed that they regularly do clerical, administrative and housekeeping work that does not require professional input. Few had

31

conducted recent activity analyses to quantify time spent on such non-nursing duties. But previous studies have found that it is common for a high proportion of nurses' time to be spent away from patients, and that between 18% and 28% of qualified nurses' time is devoted to this 'associated work' (Ref. 20). Nor is enough thought given in most hospitals to the effect on the nursing service of changing the level of provision of hospital support services. At one 500 bed hospital, the number of porters on duty during the evenings and at weekends had been reduced to two, with the result that ward cover was seriously depleted whilst nurses took urgent samples to the laboratories and collected test and X-ray results.

86. But there are marked differences of opinion about the scope for delegation under supervision of some traditional nursing duties. Although many nurses have serious doubts about the consequences for patients of relying too heavily on support workers, the extremes of opinion as to the likely eventual composition of a 'typical' acute ward team extend from:

— a 30:70 split between nurses and trained support workers, where the nurses assess, plan, supervise and evaluate patient care that is mainly delivered by support workers;

to:

— an all qualified nursing workforce with the support worker role limited to clerical work and hotel services.

(c) Confusion about Project 2000 Implementation

87. Students formed 29 per cent of the general nursing workforce in 1988, but they account for well over half of the staff available to some acute wards. Students generally perform a disproportionate amount of the direct hands-on care of patients, 45 per cent on the wards included in one research study, (Ref. 21 and 22). As Project 2000 courses start, hospitals have gradually to replace with established staff most of the contribution traditionally made by students. The number and skill mix of these replacement staff may vary markedly depending on the characteristics of each ward and the needs of its patients. Nationally, however, the overall assumption is that a fifty-fifty mix of additional basic grade staff nurses and health care support workers will initally be needed. Support workers need not necessarily directly replace students but may take over certain tasks currently performed by nurses, releasing more of their time for patient care. The new ward teams should have a lower turnover of staff and therefore be more efficient.

88. **The challenge of phased implementation:** The introduction of Project 2000 in both England and Wales is to be phased over a number of years. Hospitals studied are at various stages of planning or implementation. Welsh hospitals have had the benefit of a firm timetable. English colleges are invited to bid annually for funding. As a result, time has been wasted on nugatory planning. Some colleges have made premature changes to training intake numbers in anticipation of an increased demand for staff nurses and subsequently to build up an adequate list of applicants for the initial larger Project 2000 courses. Where acceptance of a Project 2000 funding application has been postponed, this has exacerbated difficulties in employing a cohort of newly qualifying nurses and left gaps in the projected supply of learners to the wards. Funding does not always permit temporary staff to be employed to fill these gaps. Communication between colleges (responsible for preparing course proposals and bids), personnel departments (planning support worker salary structures and roles), nurse managers (planning the deployment of

replacement staff) and the wards is often poor. There is uncertainty about timing and about the roles, capabilities and training of both support workers and Project 2000 students.

MANAGEMENT SOLUTIONS:

(a) Agreeing the Ward Staffing Needed for Quality Care

89. Injection of Project 2000 funding provides a unique opportunity to change historical patterns of ward staffing. Managers should ensure that establishments are planned in relation to agreed projections of patient activity and mix for each ward. They should set the structures within which negotiation of staffing requirements between ward sisters and their managers takes place. These structures should provide for evaluation of the effects of all changes made to staffing against specific objectives agreed with the ward sister. Evaluation should also include before and after comparison of the quality of care indicators suggested in Section 1 and of staff opinion.

90. Ward establishments should be **reviewed** annually in consultation with the ward sister, taking into account the current and prospective workload and the management responsibilities of ward staff. More frequent review may be justified if the pattern of workload on the ward varies significantly from the plan, with a change in consultant appointments, case mix or approaches to medical treatment. A zero-based review of establishments, grading and working methods should be carried out periodically.

91. An essential first step is to determine the scope for increased efficiency by examining current patterns of workload and staff utilisation through the day using **activity analysis**. This can be conducted by independent observers, but a number of hospitals have found self-recording to be both sufficiently accurate and also more likely to stimulate nurses' interest in the results and commitment to change. The activity analysis should lead to an agreed action plan for changes to working practices whose implementation should be subsequently monitored by managers. Workload assessment data should be collected at least for sample periods. The magnitude and pattern, if any, of day-by-day variation in workload should be taken into consideration, as well as the average level of workload when reviewing establishments.

92. **An agreed approach to skill mix:** Managers in some hospitals are consulting their nurses on the percentages of each type of ward activity which could be performed by health care support workers. This provides the **starting point** for negotiating the skill mix needed by each ward. Ward activity patterns are then measured and reviewed to ensure that the subsequent skill mix calculations reflect the needs of patients. It may not be appropriate for support workers to perform all the agreed activities for some patients or in some circumstances. On acute wards, workload suitable for support workers may be insufficient to justify their use on all shifts. And it will be necessary to consider whether adequate physical continuity of care can be given if the number of patient care support workers available on each shift is insufficient to assign one to each team. Such considerations could assume increasing importance with the spread of primary nursing. Ward sisters should therefore be free to change the mix of staff within agreed budgets where they can demonstrate that it is necessary for improved patient care. It is becoming increasingly common to trade 'pairs of hands' for more highly qualified staff (Ref. 23). One Grade 'D' registered nurse costs the same as 1.5 auxiliaries. An 'average' ward would need to shed about 2 posts if its sister wished to change the skill mix within its existing budget from the lowest to the highest ratio of nurses to auxiliaries observed. But managers should insist that such changes are

carefully evaluated to ensure that nurses are used appropriately and that the intended improvements in patient care are actually achieved.

(b) Support Staff:

93. Some hospitals have transferred responsibility for ward clerks from the medical records department to nursing. This has helped to ensure that the ward clerks' hours of work suit the ward and cover the peak periods for patient admissions or for telephone calls to the ward. In the absence of a ward clerk these can take up a great deal of nursing time. Some wards have extended the role of the ward clerk to include, for instance, making discharge arrangements and managing ward stationery and non clinical supplies budgets. Employment of work experience trainees to take messages and run errands can free the time of nursing staff and of ward clerks.

94. When changes are considered in portering and other support services, it is important to take into account the effect on the efficiency of nursing. Domestic support to wards needs to be available when required and under the direction of ward sisters to ensure that nurses do not spend time on domestic tasks that could be more effectively spent on patient care. The creation of posts for ward housekeepers or health care support workers mainly employed on hotel services, offers an alternative and more flexible way of relieving nurses of inappropriate domestic and ordering duties.

95. However, experience in this country and in the USA teaches that provision of extra support workers does not *automatically* lead nurses to spend a higher proportion of their time on patient related activity. Nurse managers need to pay positive attention to ways in which the ward culture can be changed and nurses given the incentive to spend more time with patients or planning care. In this way one hospital managed to reduce the proportion of qualified nurse time spent on clerical and housekeeping duties to 8%. If this level could be replicated nationally, at least £ 40 millions of nursing resources over and above the cost of employing additional clerical and domestic support could be diverted into improved patient care.

(c) Co-ordinating the introduction of Project 2000:

96. A single manager should have the responsibility of co-ordinating Project 2000 implementation including plans to introduce and train health care support workers, recruit extra nurses if required and arrangements for overcoming predicted temporary staffing deficits on the wards as learners are withdrawn. This should be done in consultation with the Director of Nursing Services, the College of Nursing, the Personnel and Finance Departments, ward sisters and their managers. All should be kept fully informed of progress, and briefed on the capabilities of each batch of Project 2000 students and support staff coming onto the ward.

Box F
IMPROVING RECRUITMENT & RETENTION

	Problems	Management solutions
(d)	Nurse wastage is too high in many hospitals.	Better analysis of reasons for sickness and why nurses leave. Surveys on staff views.
	Most nurses receive little feedback on their performance.	Recruitment, retention and return strategy. Retention targets. Extend individual performance review.
(e)	Better use could be made of remaining enrolled nurses.	Review hospital policies which restrict role of ENs.
(f)	Nurses over-involved in routine aspects of the recruitment process. Insufficient emphasis on getting the right nurse in the right job and on induction.	Improve support from personnel departments. Interview each applicant for several posts, if possible. Improve induction process; appoint mentors for new recruits.

PROBLEMS

(d) High wastage

97. High quality care is most likely to be provided by a stable and well motivated workforce. But nursing has traditionally been a *high intake, high wastage profession.* Some 20 per cent of students typically drop out during training. After qualification, although there are big regional differences in wastage rates, on average about one in seven nurses leaves the NHS each year, (Exhibit 14). The turnover of nurses in individual hospitals is significantly higher, although retention has improved during the recent period of rising unemployment. A recent report commissioned by the RCN estimates that a typical 350 bed hospital could save £ 210,000 per year if turnover was cut by 10 per cent, (Ref. 24). Stress, workloads which inhibit care and a bad atmosphere at work were named by RCN members in a 1986 survey as the three most important

Exhibit 14
MOVEMENT OF NURSES INTO AND OUT OF THE NHS
Nursing has traditionally been a high intake, high wastage profession

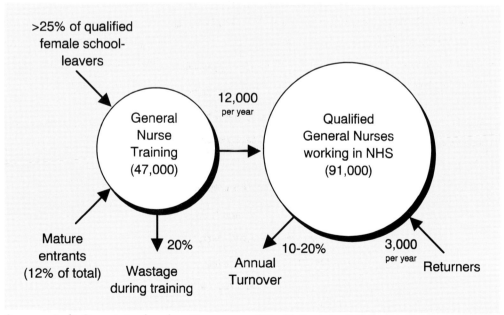

Source: *Audit Commission based on Department of Health Statistics IMS Survey Results and Project 2000 Feasibility Report.*

reasons, (Ref. 25). Nurses in the Mersey Region similarly cited inadequate staffing, the need to perform clerical and other non-nursing duties and inadequate resources as the least satisfying aspects of their job, (Ref. 26). Continued emphasis on reducing wastage and other turnover is necessary, both because of its cost and because of uncertainties about the adequacy of the future supply of nurses in some parts of the country. But not all hospitals have sufficient information on the views of nurses and why they leave to take positive measures to improve retention and target those likely to return to nursing at a later date.

98. **The Demographic Timebomb?** A high proportion of current entrants into nurse training are school leavers. Eighty eight per cent of RGNs qualify below the age of 25 years. Nationally at times over a quarter of female school leavers with five or more higher graded GCSEs up to two 'A levels' have gone into nursing (Ref. 27). The annual number of such school leavers will have fallen by 30 per cent over the decade to 1994. This has raised major concerns about whether the NHS will have an adequate supply of nurses over the coming decade. But some three quarters of the way through the period of projected decline in school leavers, hospitals taking part in the study have experienced little difficulty in staffing wards or filling planned nurse training intakes. The effects of the demographic dip have been masked in those areas which were expected to be affected most severely by the changing availability of alternative employment. Thus Project 2000 could represent a greater short-term challenge to the supply of nurses than demography.

(e) The disappearance of the enrolled nurse:

99. The potential shortfall in nursing staff could be exacerbated by the gradual disappearance under Project 2000 of enrolled nurses, one of the most stable elements of the nursing workforce. They are being encouraged to convert to registered nurse status. But many health authorities are finding it difficult to fund the full upgrading of 'C' grade junior enrolled nurse posts to 'D' grade staff nurse posts, *and* cover for current enrolled nurse posts whilst staff are on conversion courses. There are not enough places on conversion courses, and at the current rate it will take 14 years before even the current backlog of applicants is eliminated. But at present *local* policies and guidelines on what enrolled nurses may do often limit their effectiveness.

(f) Inefficient recruitment procedures

100. Responsibility for different aspects of the recruitment process is divided up in different ways in NHS hospitals, between personnel departments, nurse managers and wards. Ward sisters need to be trained in recruitment and selection, and they should then have the major say in the selection of their staff. However, it is not sensible to devote professional time to the routine administration associated with selection and recruitment, which is usually more efficiently managed by personnel departments.

MANAGEMENT SOLUTIONS
(d) Strategy for Recruitment, Retention and Return

101. In many hospitals, the current recession has temporarily diverted management attention away from the need to take measures to improve retention of nurses. In the long term, however, managers will not be able to escape a fundamental rethink of ways in which nurses' job

satisfaction can be increased through better management and changing patterns of care. A recent Kings Fund report argues that 'quick fix' solutions to improving recruitment and retention (such as provision of creches) are not sufficient and that nurses need more flexible hours and better conditions of employment (Ref. 3). It is important to achieve the right balance between the needs of the patient and the needs of the nurse. With good management these will not necessarily be incompatible. Good information on staff needs and opinions is essential. Nurse managers at a number of hospitals interview all nurses who leave in order to find out precisely why and to ensure that as many as possible consider returning if their circumstances change.

102. Senior nurses need help from personnel departments in drawing up a recruitment strategy, and in working out how to make the best use of part-time workers and job-share schemes in patient care areas. Some Regions have taken the lead in workforce planning. Mersey RHA for example has a '3Rs' strategy which sets out a framework against which hospitals can assess their staffing needs, set targets and monitor their progress towards achieving them. The best hospitals have identified their future skill needs and analysed the local consequences of Project 2000. These hospitals target their advertising, and use information from staff surveys and exit interviews to work out which supports to recruitment and retention – creches, staff accommodation, hospital transport and so on – will be the most cost-effective locally. They run 'outreach programmes' for schools, 'returners fairs', 'keep in touch' and 'update schemes' which involve periodic return visits to the hospital for nurses leaving to have families. They use the YTS scheme as a way of attracting and screening future applicants for support worker posts.

(e) The future of the enrolled nurse:

103. The rate of enrolled nurse conversion varies considerably between authorities and has been governed partly by the degree of flexibility introduced into course arrangements and timing. The current growth in distance learning may help in this respect. But in the meantime, hospitals need to review local policies restricting the role of enrolled nurses to make sure that their experience and skill is used to the maximum.

(f) Improving the Recruitment Process:

104. There is a major difference between some British and American hospitals in the emphasis placed during the recruitment process in getting the right nurse in the right job. The experience of American hospitals is that investing more time in recruitment and in induction training reduces the turnover of nurses and is cost-effective in the long term. Applicants there are frequently interviewed separately for nursing jobs on different units within the same hospital to make sure they are placed well. And, in contrast with many British hospitals where vacancy factors are imposed solely as a way of cutting budgets, at one American hospital studied, nurses are recruited *before* their predecessors leave and are then supernumerary for several weeks.

DEVELOPING CLINICAL SKILLS

105. Good quality nursing care requires not only that the staffing of wards is adequate but also that nurses are equipped with the right skills and education to adapt to modern care requirements. Chapter 1 noted the need for more professional development if primary nursing was to be implemented successfully. Each nurse should be required to keep up to date with developments in research based care and in professional thinking. Post-registration education needs should be determined systematically according to the needs of each individual nurse in relation to their post.

Box G

	Problems	Management solutions
(g)	Professional development patchy (wide variation in study days). Development needs relevant to post are seldom identified and followed up systematically.	Provide funding, time for study and opportunities for cross-fertilisation of ideas. Better use of individual performance review to identify and action needs.

PROBLEMS

(g) The need for more professional development

106. Many NHS hospitals provide insufficient opportunities for continuing professional development away from the ward. It is impossible to identify the total cost of such training and development in most hospitals since nurse training budgets cover only external courses and, of the remainder, only a proportion is provided by Colleges of Nursing. However analysis of off-duty rosters shows that the number of study and education days received by nurses once qualified is unevenly distributed and varies greatly between, and within, hospitals, (Exhibit 15). Nurses on studied wards spend an average of 6 days per year on professional development and managerial training combined compared to a public sector average of 9 days. The average for the six primary nursing wards studied was higher: 9.9 days. If the wards surveyed are typical, it would cost some £ 60 millions nationally in staff time and course expenses to bring *average* levels of post-registration nurse education up to this level on all wards.

Exhibit 15

STUDY DAYS

The number of days spent by each nurse on post-registration courses or study each year varies greatly between and within hospitals

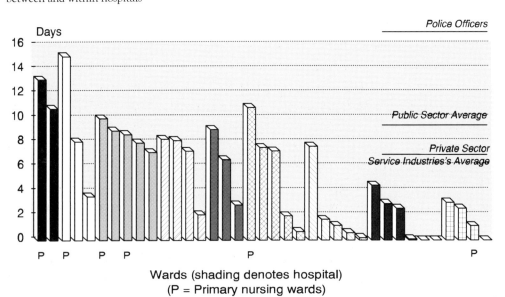

Wards (shading denotes hospital)
(P = Primary nursing wards)

Source: Audit Commission Analysis of Off-Duty Rosters

107. But post-registration study is currently confined to comparatively few individuals. Ward averages are particularly misleading where one or more nurses are granted regular day release to attend diploma or degree courses. The UKCC's proposed PREPP (post registration education and practice project) scheme would require all nurses to undergo a minimum of five days' further professional training every three years to maintain their registration. Unless available time and funds are distributed more equitably, even this would represent a major increase in training which will need to be properly funded. At present many hospitals have long waiting lists for certain internal courses. And nurses are often expected to bear a portion of the costs of attending any external courses. Control of training and development budgets in most NHS hospitals is highly centralised because they are too small to be fragmented. Each floor (ward) sister at a private hospital studied controlled a bigger budget for external courses (£ 4,000) than that for the whole of one 250 bed NHS hospital despite equally good access to internal courses.

108. **Training Support Workers:** The work of most ward auxiliaries reflects the length of their nursing experience and the confidence of the ward sister in their abilities more than any formal qualification. This creates difficulties for the ward if the nurse in charge does not have prior knowledge or personal experience of the individual on which to base her judgement about how much she can delegate safely. It is also problematic for the auxiliary when she wishes to move to another post and has no objective proof of the extent of her capabilities. The introduction of health care assistants under Project 2000 was intended to end these uncertainties by setting out universally recognised lists of core competencies and attainment, subject to examination. But at the time of publication, uncertainty about training for health care support workers persists. It is understood that the national system of vocational training under the auspices of the NCVQ will not be mandatory, and so the difficulties for individuals changing employer may remain. Agreement of required competencies has lagged behind the withdrawal of nursing students on traditional courses from some wards. In consequence some, but not all, authorities have instituted their own unrecognised local training schemes for level 1 and forward planning of skill mix has been inhibited.

MANAGEMENT SOLUTIONS
(g) Improving Post-Registration Education and Training
109. Many nurses believe in-service training on up-to-date research based treatment methods is cost-effective. They claim that it is possible to reduce lengths of stay and expenditure on treatments now considered ineffective. At one NHS hospital studied individual performance reviews of all nurses are used to identify staff development needs systematically. These are incorporated into a planned programme. In this way, decisions are taken by a manager who knows the training and development needs of each nurse in relation to her post. These can then be married with individual aspirations. Training records are kept and used to ensure that opportunities are allocated equitably. Another hospital has developed a computer programme to keep track of course attendance and requests.

110. **Training for Support Staff:** The needs of ward support staff for in-post training should also be reviewed annually. Where appropriate, this training should lead to a recognised qualification or certificate. Support staff should not be required to perform duties for which they have not been trained.

MAKING BEST DAY-TO-DAY USE OF WARD STAFF

111. Making best use of nurses involves balancing the sometimes conflicting objectives of ensuring that the number and mix of staff available on each shift reflect workload and of preserving, as far as is possible, continuity of care to patients.

Box H

Nurses are not used well:

(h)	Shift patterns and overlaps are inappropriate to patient needs.	Educate sisters and give them freedom to negotiate new shift patterns appropriate to ward workload. Help them to overcome barriers to change. Encourage review of activity in the afternoon shift overlap period.
(i)	Poor Rostering.	Provide training on good rostering which preserves continuity of care. Periodic management audit of efficiency, effectiveness, equity.

Response to mismatches between staff and workload is often inappropriate.

(j)	Confused objectives for workload assessment:- Excessive staff movement is inefficient, bad for morale and disrupts continuity.	Concentrate on using workload assessment to help nurses pace their work better. Move nurses only as a last resort, involving sisters in the decision.
	Nurses have insufficient control over their workload.	Facilitate doctor/nurse agreement on circumstances and procedures for restricting ward workload if insoluble shortages of nurses occur over a sustained period.
(k)	Bank/agency nurses are often employed to 'make up the numbers' regardless of workload, in a way which disrupts continuity of care, and may work below the grade at which they are paid.	More flexible rostering of ward staff is an alternative. Workload assessment and delegated budgets improve control over use of temporary staff. Restrict nurses to wards with which they are familiar. Better induction for bank nurses.

PROBLEMS:
NURSES ARE NOT USED WELL IN RELATION TO PATIENT NEEDS
(h) Shift patterns and overlaps

112. The origin of the shift patterns worked on many wards is historical. Research has concentrated on the effects on quality of care and on staff of such major changes as changing from three to two shifts per day, (Ref. 28). But at local level, there have been comparatively few attempts to evaluate the costs and benefits of different shift patterns.

113. Previous studies have highlighted the potential benefits of shorter afternoon shift overlaps. The National Audit Office in its 1985 report commented that in a general hospital of 450 to 500 beds, their cost could equate to that of 40 to 50 whole-time nurses (Ref. 17). Some hospitals have reduced these overlaps considerably by shortening night shifts or changing daytime shift patterns. But the length and use of afternoon shift overlaps still varies markedly, from three quarters of an hour to over four hours (including an unpaid meal break) in hospitals studied, and sometimes between similar wards in the same hospitals (Exhibit 16).

Exhibit 16
LENGTH OF AFTERNOON SHIFT-OVERLAP
The length and use of shift-overlaps varies markedly between hospitals

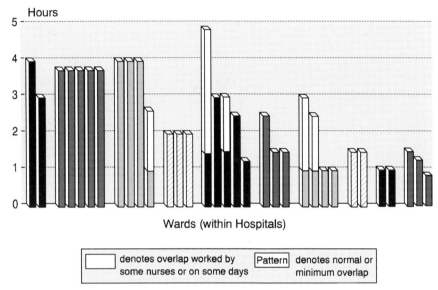

Note: *Not all staff work the full overlap*
Source: *Audit Commission Study Sites*

114. Although many ward sisters have the authority to vary shift patterns, very few have had management training to help them use their power constructively and only a minority have done so. Long overlaps are not *necessarily* inefficient if used for the benefit of patients, but activity analyses rarely demonstrate any increase in direct patient care at this time. Not all staff nurses favour them. To quote one:

> 'The overlap is frustrating. One person thinks the other is doing something, so it is missed. Patients see nurses floating around doing odd jobs. If you are on a late you have to wait for the early staff to go before you can get your own jobs done.'

Revision of shift times, with the agreement of ward staff could often release resources which could be used to improve ward cover and overall patient care.

(i) Rostering
115. Staffing and skill-mix differences are even greater from day to day and between shifts on the same ward than between similar wards, (Exhibit 17, overleaf). On one ward, the number of qualified nurses on the early shift varied from one to six. The skill mix on four successive Saturdays ranged between 16 and 50 per cent qualified. This degree of variation is typical of many of the wards studied. Although some of it reflects anticipated workload, days when the ward is 'on take' for emergency admissions or on 'theatre days', staffing variations frequently bear little relation to changes in ward occupancy or patient care needs.

Exhibit 17
DAY TO DAY STAFFING OF WARDS
Staffing and skill-mix differences from day to day are even greater than those between similar wards

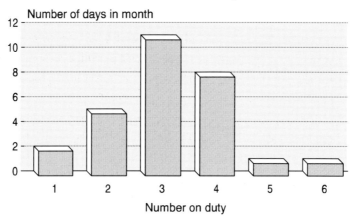

Staff Present on the Early Shift

4 Mondays   4 Thursdays   4 Saturdays

RGNs   ENs   Auxiliaries   Learners

Qualified Nurses on Early Shift

Number of days in month

Number on duty

Source: Audit Commission analysis of nursing rosters for four weeks in September

116. Variations in cover and skill-mix on the planned 'off-duty' roster may reflect practical constraints on scheduling nurses. The current fluctuating availability of 'learners' is a particular problem, (Exhibit 18). A recent study conducted over a 40 week period on one ward showed that the ward received the agreed number of learners for only 4 weeks (Ref. 12). It was understaffed for 26 weeks and overstaffed for the remaining ten. The additional supervisory burden makes too many learners on the ward as difficult to manage as a shortage of staff.

117. Few ward sisters give priority to continuity of patient care when drawing up 'off-duties'. As a result they are unable to organise care in a consistent way. Nurses frequently have to help out other teams, caring for patients whom they do not know. Even where adequate staffing of each team on each shift has been arranged, it may be upset by temporary transfers of staff to other wards.

Exhibit 18
ALLOCATION OF 'LEARNERS' TO A 28 BED MEDICAL WARD OVER A 40 WEEK PERIOD
Marked variation from week to week in the number of 'learners' available to wards causes problems

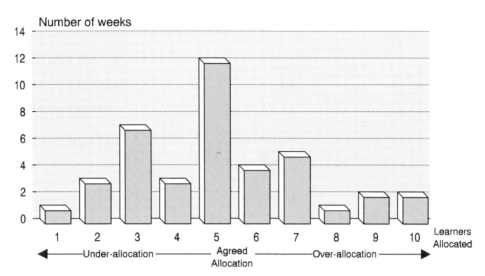

Source: Data gathered by S.Procter (Ref.12)

118. Some sisters appear to pay excessive attention to staff preferences when constructing the roster. Clearly 'requests' should be met as far as possible if it helps maintain morale, but sisters on some wards listed these as the prime consideration when constructing rosters. In a few wards, higher grade nurses appear to work a disproportionate number of weekends and evenings. Because of the special duty payments involved, this should be avoided unless it is required to meet the needs of the patient or for effective management of the hospital and nurse workforce.

Inappropriate response to mismatches between staff and workload

119. Actual ward cover is affected by staff sickness, and unforeseen circumstances such as provision of patient escorts or movement of nurses to help out other wards. If the number of nurses available on a shift is judged to be insufficient for the workload, nurse managers try to move nurses from other apparently overstaffed wards or authorise the employment of bank and agency staff. Both can be bad for continuity of care, especially on wards practising primary nursing.

(j) Use made of workload assessment

120. Many systems, both manual and computerised, have been developed to assess and project the numbers and mix of nurses required on a ward as an aid to deploying available staff where they are most likely to be needed. Objectives for workload assessment are frequently confused, and installed systems have often produced a mass of data but little improvement. A common assumption by managers is that they will be able to use the information to move nurses from one ward to another to improve the match between staff and workload. But if the planned disposition of the ward team is frequently disrupted by temporary transfers or by importation of staff who are not fully familiar with the ward, both efficiency and the quality of patient care given is likely to suffer. Borrowed staff are unlikely to know the patients and will not be committed to

the same ward ethos. For these reasons, many American hospitals have now abandoned large pools of nurses who could be moved around the hospital in favour of measures to encourage stability in ward teams.

121. The usefulness of workload assessment systems has also been limited by the inability of nurses to project with sufficient accuracy both the number of patients likely to be present on a ward from day to day, and the average workload associated with each of them. This is particularly the case on medical wards where some 90 per cent of patients are emergency admissions. And data often does not arrive in time for managers to take appropriate action. Nurses have insufficient control over their own workload to enable them to maintain standards of care over sustained periods of mismatch between staff availability and patients' needs. But only a minority of those hospitals that collect data use it to trigger reductions in nursing workload in such circumstances. Care suffers accordingly.

(k) Use made of bank and agency nurses:

122. Few sisters have sufficient staff of their own or short term flexibility in the way they are rostered to cover all gaps in the roster resulting from staff sickness or planned absences. Gaps are therefore typically filled using part-time nurses employed on the hospital's 'bank'. Employment of temporary nurses supplied by private agencies is less significant nationally, but consumes up to 17 per cent of expenditure on nursing within some districts in South East England. At one hospital studied, bank staff have to be 'ordered' one week in advance. They can therefore be utilised only to cover those staff shortages that are predictable. Once booked, it is not customary for bank and agency nurses to be cancelled. They are frequently used to 'make up the numbers' on a ward, regardless of potential workload or whether it is necessary for patient care. Conversely at only one hospital studied are ward sisters permitted to book bank nurses purely because *workload* is exceptionally heavy.

123. If large numbers of different temporary nurses are employed on each ward and no specific induction training is given, their presence is disruptive to continuity of care and imposes a considerable additional burden on permanent staff. There are marked differences in practice with regard to the care exercised in obtaining temporary staff who are familiar with the layout and procedures of the ward, or even with care of the type of patients treated on it. One unit even has a policy that the same agency nurse may not be employed on a single ward for more than three consecutive days. A ward attempting to introduce primary nursing was allocated 47 *different* temporary nurses over a one month period. Their lack of familiarity with the ward means that agency staff are often allocated work below the grade at which they are employed. Added to the uncertainties of a fluctuating workload, the ward sister never knows precisely what skills will be available for deployment on each shift.

MANAGEMENT SOLUTIONS
(h) Shift patterns which meet the needs of patients

124. Managers should encourage ward sisters to change shift patterns within existing budgets to match patient needs and make best use of available staff. Some have already done this. But the majority will need more training on the possibilities of change and help in analysing implications for costs and organisation of care. Regulations may need to be changed to permit more flexibility in the number of hours that a nurse is rostered to work during each individual pay period, so that for instance shifts do not always sum to exactly 75 hours every fortnight. Where shifts have been reviewed, numbers and skill-mix of staff available at key times of day have been improved. Part-time staff can be used to cover times of the day when demand for routine care is greatest. Communication is better. Time has been made available for on the ward teaching and seminars and for attendance at standard setting groups, management groups and professional forums. Managers should be encouraging nurses to think more about whether long shift overlaps every day are the best way to accommodate activities such as instruction of learners, completion of documentation and occasional management meetings (Exhibit 19, overleaf). Changing the overlap times can have a beneficial effect on the length of the night shift or reduce the length of day shifts. *If the sites studied are typical, reduction of the afternoon overlap to a maximum of one hour throughout the country could theoretically, even after abolition of unpaid meal breaks, release nursing resources costing some £50 millions for redeployment to times when patient needs are greater.*

125. Timing of staff child care, transport and catering facilities can be very real constraints to changing established shift patterns but, once these have been identified as problems, many can be addressed by management. Any savings that would result from changes to shift times should be taken into consideration when evaluating the cost-effectiveness of schemes such as providing hospital transport or extending the hours of creches.

(i) More efficient and effective rostering of staff

126. A good roster should be efficient, equitable so as to foster good staff morale and effective in providing adequate ward cover and continuity of care. It needs to reflect the chosen form of organisation. Thus many wards operating team or primary nursing initially construct a separate 'off-duty' for each team. These are then combined and adjusted if necessary. In this way the number of different nurses caring for the patient during his stay in hospital is kept to the minimum. The roster should be prepared well in advance so that staff can fit other engagements around their work commitments. In this way the need for last minute changes, which often disrupt the planned organisation of care, should be minimised. Managers should ensure that adequate training on all these aspects is provided. The potential of computerised rostering systems for enabling alternative rosters to be costed and examined has not yet been fully realised. Periodic management audits of rosters should also be carried out.

(j) Systematic collection and use of workload assessment data

127. All wards should operate a systematic method for timely measurement of current and, where feasible, prospective nurse workload. A subsequent report on use of nursing management systems will consider practical aspects. None of the available methods is theoretically perfect but, if used well, any could help to improve consistency of care. The process of installing such systems, whether computerised or manual, can in itself heighten nurses' awareness of the way they use their time and of how they interact with patients. Workload data should not be used mechanistically but, together with professional judgement, it can improve planning and inform decisions about allocation of patients to nurses and about the levels and mix of ward staffing needed on each shift to maintain agreed standards.

Exhibit 19
USE OF THE SHIFT-OVERLAP
Is this long shift-overlap really necessary

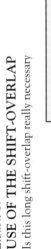

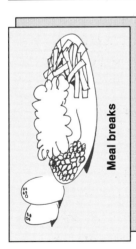

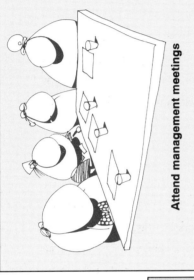

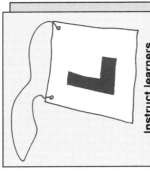

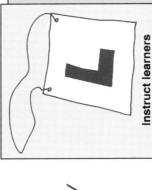

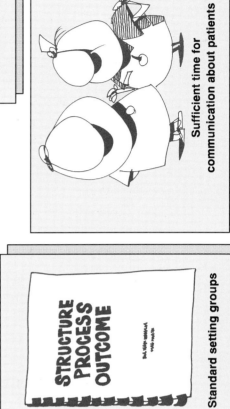

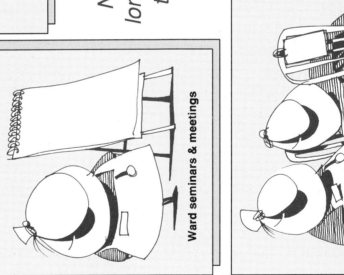

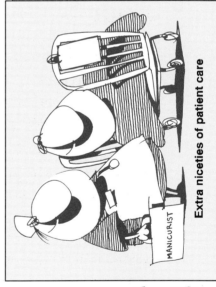

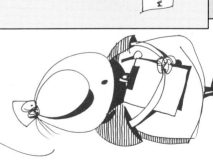

Nurses should consider whether long shift overlaps are the best way to accommodate such activities

Source: Audit Commission

128. The Clinical Management Group of one surgical unit in the study sample agrees every year the expected workload of each ward and the parameters that constitute 'exceptional' daily workloads. If these parameters are exceeded, ward sisters have delegated authority to order bank or agency staff at short notice, and, conversely, if the workload falls below the minimum, the ward sister will offer staff for redeployment to other wards. Managers at another hospital stress the importance of involving ward sisters fully in day to day decisions about any staff movements. Management training for ward sisters helps to ensure that such decisions are taken on a rational but sensitive basis. Some hospitals carry out periodic surveys of sisters' opinions on standards of care and on the adequacy of staffing levels on specific shifts.

129. Where there are not enough staff to cope with the workload it may be necessary to make difficult decisions about restricting less urgent admissions, discharging convalescent patients early or moving patients to other less appropriate wards. Two hospitals out of ten in the study had closed beds during a period of high staff sickness, and another had temporarily changed the allocation of new patients to wards so as to restrict workloads. Nurses need to participate in decisions about admissions (numbers and case-mix), discharges and transfers to and from wards and be involved with managers and clinicians in discussing the implications for quality of patient care.

(k) Supplementing ward staffing

130. **More flexible rostering:** A major teaching hospital is attempting to improve the match of daily staffing to workload by asking nurses to be more flexible about which shifts they work. Nurses specify which extra shifts they would be prepared to work and days when they would like additional time off. They are contacted by telephone and asked to change shifts if workload is unexpectedly high or low. Split shifts are not involved. Preliminary indications are that most nurses like the scheme. Such arrangements are common in private hospitals and in the USA. It is uncommon for nurses to be paid overtime, but some hospitals have found that it is preferable to cover periods of peak workload shorter than a full shift in this way, rather than increasing establishments or employing bank staff for a full shift.

131. **Better use of temporary nurses:** The value of delegated staff budgets in ensuring that bank and agency staff are used only when justified by workload is discussed in Section 3. But a number of hospitals have found that efficiency and quality of care is improved if employment of individual bank nurses is restricted to a small number of wards with which they are familiar. Some have set up separate nurse banks for each clinical directorate. A private hospital studied uses a higher ratio of bank to permanent staff than is common in NHS hospitals and is more prescriptive about when they must be available for work. Their bank staff are supernumerary during the induction period and subsequently participate fully alongside permanent staff in training. This mirrors practice in the best American Hospitals. One studied has a separate bank for each "floor" (equivalent to a ward) and will only employ on a 'per-diem' basis nurses who have previously worked full-time on that floor.

3. Managing the Nursing Service

132. The management of hospital nursing has been in a state of flux for some years. The general trend has been gradually to replace 1970's 'consensus management' and the tiered management structures recommended in the Salmon Report with Griffiths-style 'general management'. Many hospitals are now moving towards more decentralised management by clinical teams. This section examines key features that differentiate 'traditional' and 'progressive' structures and styles of nursing management. On the ground, nursing management does not conform in a straightforward or simple way to either stereotype – most hospitals contain some elements of both. Nursing management varies immensely, in structure, in style, and in operational matters from one hospital to another. No single 'solution' or pace of change is right for all hospitals. But whichever path is chosen will need to promote the ideal of clinically relevant management led by patient needs. This requires strong leadership, good communication and a well educated nursing work-force.

STYLES OF MANAGEMENT

Box 1

	Problems	Management solutions
(a)	Lack of clinical focus in management. Insufficient devolution of responsibility to ward sisters.	Clinically based middle nurse management. Devolve to wards: – day-to-day budget management – flexibility (skill mix/shifts) – staff recruitment. Prepare / train ward sisters for extended management role.

(a) Lack of clinical focus in nurse management

133. **Some** nurse managers interviewed during the study see their main function in terms of **'solving staffing problems'**. Much of this work is reactive and involves moving nurses around the hospital to even out staff shortages. Many of them seem to devote a great deal of their time to individual nurses: policing their absences, behaviour and dress, and authorising training requests on an ad hoc basis. The nurses whom they manage typically say that they receive little feedback on their performance except when things go wrong. Other studies suggest that such feelings are widespread, one reporting that of 177 sisters interviewed, 70 per cent suffered stress because they received feedback only when their performance was seen as unsatisfactory (Ref. 29). These managers may also spend a lot of time on administration: compiling sickness returns, completing orders for temporary staff, and bed state returns. Some hospitals also have senior nurses without line management responsibilities who are entirely engaged on such administration, much of it repetitive low-grade clerical work. Such nurse managers may describe themselves as 'keeping an eye on the budget', but typically they do not actively participate in the budget setting process, nor do they have authority to vire between budget heads. Their management of the budget is therefore limited to restricting authorisation of bank staff if it is overspent.

134. These 'traditional' nurse managers generally appear to refer most decisions about the nursing **service** up the management hierarchy. This can have a stifling effect if, for instance, wards want to experiment with different shift times. But although they retain strict control over nursing **staff** and their deployment, many nurse managers regard day to day decisions about **patient care** as the preserve of the ward sister. They say that they supervise the quality of nursing care by 'visiting the wards', sometimes up to three times a day. Their ward nurses typically refer to this as 'checking up on them'. A number of those interviewed commented that, at the end of such a visit, they are not necessarily clear as to its purpose or whether the ward has passed or failed in the manager's judgement. Many managers 'lend a hand' when wards are busy. Such help may be appreciated but, because the managers' time is short and they do not know the patients, they tend to help out with tasks such as making beds, drug rounds or handing out patient meals. In other words, they are used in much the same way as temporary staff on the ward.

135. Such managers' lack of clinical focus may be reflected in the way some of their sisters manage their wards, concentrating on administration and helping out when there is a shortage of staff to the exclusion of real involvement with patients or in developing care. In most hospitals, both ward sisters and nurse managers receive little preparation for their new responsibilities. And those responsibilities are often not matched with delegated powers, for budget management or for staff recruitment and deployment.

MANAGEMENT SOLUTIONS
(a) Nurse managers who 'develop the service'

136. Other nurse managers see their job as **'developing the nursing service'** rather than 'managing nurses'. Many of these have replaced the ad-hoc policing and monitoring activities associated with traditional nurse management with more systematic approaches. Thus they use individual performance review (IPR) to set objectives for the wards and identify staff development needs. Many have set up systems to collect data on the quality of care rather than relying solely on their own subjective impressions. Many are actively involved in budget setting and use such control as they may have over budgets to shape the service. However they delegate day-to-day decisions about resource use, as much as possible, to ward sisters. They emphasise good communication between managers and staff. They encourage innovation and make themselves available to discuss changes and ideas. They facilitate the spread of successful innovation to other wards. Although they are usually well known to the nursing staff, if they visit the wards it is for an explicit purpose – to discuss changes, or give guidance and advice.

137. Under managers of this second type, the role of ward sisters is changing in a way consistent with the recommendations of Section 1. They devote more time to managing and developing ward staff rather than involving themselves in decisions about the day- to-day care

Exhibit 20
CONTRASTING SYLES OF MANAGEMENT
Some nurse managers only see their function as solving staffing problems but others emphasise service development

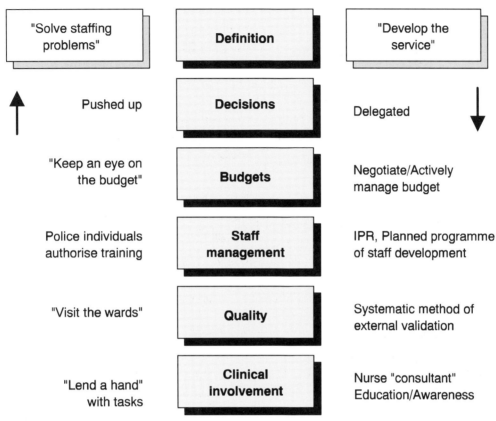

"Solve staffing problems"	**Definition**	"Develop the service"
↑ Pushed up	**Decisions**	Delegated ↓
"Keep an eye on the budget"	**Budgets**	Negotiate/Actively manage budget
Police individuals authorise training	**Staff management**	IPR, Planned programme of staff development
"Visit the wards"	**Quality**	Systematic method of external validation
"Lend a hand" with tasks	**Clinical involvement**	Nurse "consultant" Education/Awareness

Source: Audit Commission

of individual patients. Thus management is more clinically based and focused on using resources and developing nursing to give better care to patients, (Exhibit 20).

138. **Preparing nurses for management** Progressive nurse management can best be spread by placing greater emphasis on the preparation of nurses for their new management roles. In America it is common for each new 'head nurse' (sister) or manager to have a preceptor for some months after her appointment. And in France, leading hospitals expect nurses to attend a nine month management course at the 'Ecole des Cadres' before they are appointed to the post of surveillante, the ward sister's French equivalent. A standard block of classroom training prior to taking up post along the French model may not be the most appropriate way to prepare British nurses, but there is a need to acknowledge formally the needs of newly appointed sisters for management development and support, and to establish formal mechanisms to meet them. Ward sisters and clinical nurse managers should have access to management courses on terms equal to that of other middle managers in the hospital.

Box J

	Problems	Management solutions
Management without information:-		
(b)	Poor data on cost of ward resources and inadequate training on meaningful use of such information.	Improve financial systems to permit devolved budgetary control. Provide training and support.
(c)	Slow takeup of nurse management systems (NMS).	Prioritise computerisation of patient information required by nurses. Clarify objectives of NMS and 'model' its use. Provide adequate training on system potential as well as support.

PROBLEMS:

(b) Inadequate Systems for Management of Financial Resources

139. The annual nursing budget in a 500 bed district general hospital was some £7.5 millions in 1990/91, a third of total costs. A 26 bed ward would typically have a budget of around £250,000, although the content and structure of these budgets can vary considerably. About 85 per cent of that is for the pay of directly employed nurses. Ten per cent is for supplies. But in the past most nurses have received only patchy and often inaccurate information on the major costs of the resources that they control.

140. **Problems in devolving budgetary responsibility:** Although increasingly hospitals plan to devolve both pay and non-pay budgets to the wards, many are experiencing difficulty. In some, it is the financial system that is the problem – not all financial systems break expenditure down to ward level. In others, it is the management process that is at odds with the principles behind devolution. In some hospitals, for example, even though there has been devolution, budget managers are not properly consulted when budgets are set, or the budgets include items over which they have no control. Most hospitals retain centrally managed budgets for continuing education and for the employment of bank and agency nurses. They also hold on centrally to the refunds of statutory maternity pay and statutory sickness benefit, so that the ward sister, who needs to cover the shortfall, is not able to exercise full control over the ward's resource. Likewise, the funds that should be transferred from Schools of Nursing to the wards when the supply of learners to wards falls below agreed levels are usually retained centrally.

(c) Slow take-up of nurse management systems

141. The main building blocks of nurse management systems (workload assessment, possibly linked to care plans, and rostering) were discussed in Section Two. In the NHS, the take-up of computerised systems has been comparatively slow, despite the financial incentives that have been made available, and good use has not always been made of the information generated. The companion paper on effective use of nurse management systems and establishment setting methodologies examines reasons why. There has often been over-concentration on systems which promise time savings for nurses and managers rather than systems which improve the quality of care.

(b) Better financial systems and devolved budgetary control

142. The limited experience to date of budgetary devolution to wards confirms that it helps to ensure that staff are allocated sensibly in relation to the workload. Although ward sisters who do not manage their own financial budgets often say that they have neither the time, the training nor the inclination to do so, the experience of American hospitals suggests that they may change their minds. American nurses had similar reservations a decade ago, but head nurses (the equivalent of the ward sister) now appear convinced that it is to their advantage to have full control over their own resources. American hospitals put great effort into training and day-to-day support in the preparation and monitoring of budgets. They also monitor expenditure carefully through computer terminals on each 'floor'. Nurses are encouraged to feel that accountants are there to give constructive help rather than to rap them over the knuckles if overspends occur. Those hospitals studied are currently moving away from fixed yearly budgets and working towards flexible budgets linked to activity.

143. One NHS hospital in the Audit Commission sample is well on the way towards devolved budgets. Ward sisters control the pay budgets and are responsible for the costs of bank and agency staff. As a result, the sisters have started to cancel temporary staff when the workload does not justify their employment, and buy them in when it does. The wards gain financial credits when they lend staff, and debits when they borrow from other wards. There is less movement of staff between wards, but greater willingness to lend assistance when it is called for. As an incentive, all the wards within a clinical group are permitted to share their savings and spend them on ward improvements.

(c) Nurse Management Systems

144. Despite the reservations expressed about their present use in some hospitals, computerised systems will, if the current pitfalls can be overcome, offer the potential of improved financial management and better information for patient care. American research suggests that it is more cost-effective to concentrate initially on improving the information available to nurses about patients, than on computer systems for managing nurses (Ref. 30). It is also vital that nurses and managers receive adequate training and support, not only in how to operate systems, but also in how to use them to explore better ways of providing care. The companion paper reviews strengths and weaknesses of presently available systems, and draws general lessons from study hospitals on best practice in their use, implementation, and the support required.

CHOOSING AN APPROPRIATE NURSING MANAGEMENT STRUCTURE
Box K

	Problems	Management solutions
(d)	There are too many nurse managers in some hospitals.	Many hospitals could reduce nurse management costs to 2% of the pay bill without sacrificing quality (potential national saving £35m).
(e)	Responsibilities are often confused and leadership is lacking.	Clarify responsibilities.
		DNS/Matron to give professional leadership (strategy, practice development, education, sit on management board) but not to manage nurses/nursing budgets.

PROBLEMS

(d) How much management is needed?

145. Nursing management structures and their associated costs vary greatly between hospitals. At hospitals in the Audit Commission sample, the costs of nurse managers and senior nurses who do not have regular day to day contact with patients range from just 0.6 per cent to 7.1 per cent of the nursing pay budget, a twelvefold variation, (Exhibit 21). This comparison does not take into account the differing opportunity costs of greater delegation of management responsibilities to the wards, or consequent variations in the workload of personnel and other directorates. It does include the cost of any time which general managers estimate that they spend

Exhibit 21
NURSING MANAGEMENT COSTS
Nursing management costs vary between 0.6 and 7.1% of nursing pay budgets

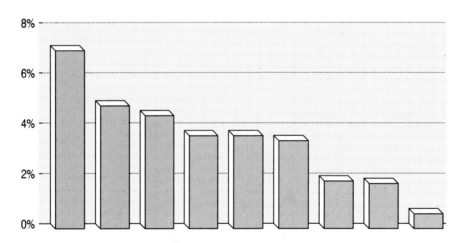

Note: Management costs include pay of general managers involved in day-to-day nurse management and of senior nurses who do not have regular direct contact with patients.

Source: Audit Commission Site Visits

on traditional nursing management functions.

146. Four of the ten hospitals studied retain a traditional 'pyramid' nurse management structure of the type developed in most hospitals during the 1970s following the Salmon Report.

In one site visited, the Director of Nursing Services (DNS) reports to the Unit General Manager (UGM), but in all other respects management of the nursing service is distinct from that of support services and the rest of the hospital. The UGM is thus the lowest level of manager empowered to take decisions on all the nursing, housekeeping and support services provided on a ward. There are two levels of nurse manager (CNM), some with only two people reporting to them, between the Director of Nursing Services and ward sisters (Exhibit 22). Nurse management costs at this

Exhibit 22
NURSING MANAGEMENT STRUCTURES (1)
Four of the ten hospitals studied retain a traditional 'pyramid' management structure

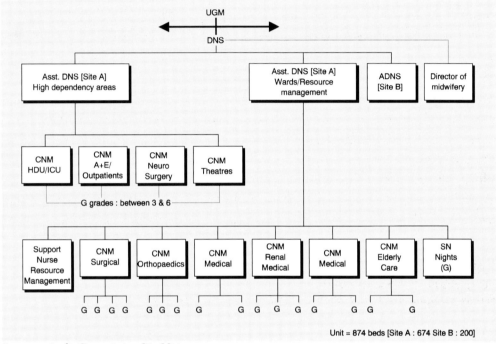

Source: Audit Commission Site Visits

hospital are 3.4% of the nursing pay budget.

147. In contrast, at the hospital with the cheapest nursing management of those studied ward sisters report directly to the hospital manager, a former matron. Similar flat structures exist within clinical directorates in some larger hospitals. They are not necessarily synonymous with general as opposed to functional management of nursing.

148. The traditional 'solving staffing problems' style of management is also more common at those hospitals studied which have pyramids of nurse management, especially where managers have a relatively small span of control. In contrast, at hospitals with flatter structures, wards tend to be more self sufficient with less day to day movement of staff between them. However at some hospitals where there are no nurse managers, although good ward sisters may feel that they have more freedom to innovate, the less experienced may be left behind.

149. **Senior nurse posts:** Many hospitals have created development posts for senior nurses in quality assurance, professional development, resource management or computing. These posts can contribute very positively to the development of nursing, but they need to be filled by enthusiasts with appropriate backgrounds, training and experience. A number of hospitals have used this type of post as homes for displaced senior staff and nurse managers close to retirement. Some individuals have adapted well, but many have neither the aptitude nor the inclination for their new jobs.

(e) Confused Responsibilities:

150. At several hospitals studied nurse managers' roles have been changed without proper definition or agreement of the scope of their new responsibilities. At one, following management reorganisation, some nurse managers were left with budgetary responsibilities for wards they did not control, whilst others were responsible for wards for which they did not hold the budget. This confused 'interim' situation prevailed for some considerable time.

151. **Divided management responsibility for day and night nurses**: The way night nursing staff are managed illustrates widespread confusion of responsibility at ward level. Theoretically, all 'G' grade sisters have *24 hour responsibility* for their wards. But in five out of the ten hospitals studied, it is not clear who is responsible for the care patients receive at night because the hospital also has a night nurse manager and the sister has no say over how the ward is staffed at night. In many hospitals, night staff are moved around the hospital and there is no attempt to keep them on the same wards each week. Even where internal rotation of shifts has been introduced, experienced staff nurses may be redeployed from their own wards by night managers to supervise bank and agency staff, use of which is particularly high at night. Clearly this has an adverse effect on continuity of planned care as well as on the promotion of clear responsibility.

MANAGEMENT SOLUTIONS
(d) Lean but effective management structures

152. An increasing number of hospitals have replaced one tier of nurse management with a senior ward sister post at 'H' or 'I' grade within each clinical unit, (Exhibit 23). As well as running their own ward, these senior sisters act as 'consultants' to other wards within their unit, thus overcoming many of the deficiencies of very flat management structures. By retaining a real hands-on clinical role, senior sisters are generally perceived by ward nurses as having more clinical credibility than the nurse managers, clinical or otherwise, that they superseded. And the changes should allow administrative as well as clinical decisions to take place closer to the patient. Such structures fit well with clinical directorates where these have been introduced.

153. They also have financial advantages. At one hospital with this type of structure, management costs amount to only 1.8% of the nursing pay budget. If the Audit Commission sample of hospitals is typical, and if management costs could be reduced everywhere to a maximum of two per cent of the nursing pay budget, some **£35 millions** of nursing expenditure would be released for other priorities.

(e) Strong Leadership – Bring back the Matron?

154. Every Directly Managed Unit or Self Governing Trust needs a recognisable professional head of nursing services responsible for service strategy and for policy on practice development and education. The importance of the nursing component in patient care makes it essential for that person to sit on the Management Board. Some trusts are creating a 'Matron' post to fill this role. The Matron of the 1990s though must be the head *of the nursing service* rather

Exhibit 23
NURSING MANAGEMENT STRUCTURES (2)
An increasing number of hospitals have replaced one tier of nurse management with a senior ward sister within each clinical unit

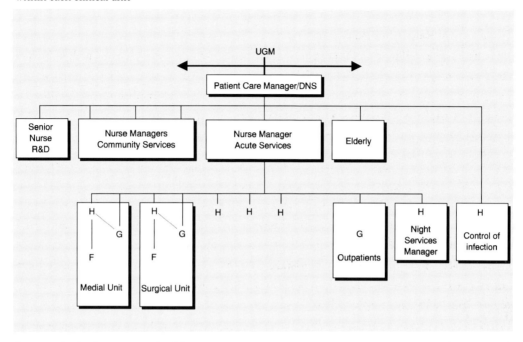

Source: Audit Commission Site Visit

than the line manager *of the nurses*. It is important not to create a post at odds with decentralisation and devolution of budgets to clinical directorates and wards.

STRATEGY

155. **A common vision:** Nursing is too important a component of patient care and consumes and controls too large a proportion of hospital resources, to be left to develop in isolation or as an afterthought to clinical reorganisation. The commitment of the whole of the hospital and unit management team to a common vision of the way nursing should develop is necessary for improvements in patient care and effective use of nurses. The best way to achieve this commitment is for nurses to take the lead and, with general managers and clinicians, jointly to develop a comprehensive nursing strategy.

Box K

	Problems	Management solutions
(f)	Lack of strategic vision for the nursing service. Rushed and uncoordinated change. Insufficient interface between nursing and the rest of hospital management.	A nursing strategy flowing from analysis of future patient needs and linked to hospital plans. Integrate nursing developments with those elsewhere in the hospital so nursing reflects changes in management and medical practice.

PROBLEMS

(f) Lack of Strategic Vision

156. **What happened to the Strategy for Nursing?** In 1989 the Department of Health published *its* 'Strategy for Nursing', (reference 31). It suggested 44 targets for action to improve nursing practice, availability of 'manpower', education, leadership and management. Managers and staff in all health care settings were asked to set timetables for implementation. But locally, only one hospital in the study has agreed a comprehensive local strategy for its nursing services, in most others, plans are fragmented. At the majority of hospitals, change in the nursing service has largely been reactive. It has not flowed from a clear idea about what nursing is, where it should be heading, or the structural changes needed to support its development. Communication between different parts of the nursing service within the same district is often poor. Nurses on the wards, and even managers above them, are often, for instance, not aware of the latest initiatives in the School of Nursing.

157. **Uncoordinated Change:** Over the past decade, nurse managers and nurses in every hospital in the Audit Commission sample have had to contend with major change in almost every aspect of their work. Some of the changes originate within nursing. As noted above, in many hospitals, the preparations for project 2000 have made the size of the student cohorts coming on to the wards unpredictable and subject to change. The mentorship role of first level registered nurses has been extended to include continuous assessment of students, and simultaneously, the same nurses have often been expected to become involved in the assessment of support staff (nursing auxiliaries and health care support workers) on the ward. Other changes affecting nursing services have their roots elsewhere. First general management, and then the reorganisation of management at sub-unit level into clinical management groups, have had a fundamental impact on nursing management structures. Amalgamations and closures of wards have meant that nurses used to patients in one clinical specialty have had to work with different types of patients and clinical conditions without proper preparation. Nurses have had to learn how to use information technology introduced on to many wards to assist with workload assessment, rosters and care planning. In many hospitals managers have found it difficult to co-ordinate the number and control the pace of change impacting on nursing.

MANAGEMENT SOLUTIONS

(f) Developing a strategy

158. A coherent nursing strategy, agreed by a cross-section of nurses, should help to avoid some of the problems associated with unplanned and uncoordinated change. It offers a framework within which each proposed change in the service can be tested, and, as decentralisation of management becomes more common, it will allow a consistent view about nursing services to be taken across the hospital. Within the framework of a strategy, it should be possible to decide priorities and ensure that the pace of change is manageable with a timetable and resources that allow for subsequent evaluation.

159. A nursing strategy should take an analysis of the needs of patients and their families as its point of departure. Needs change over time in line with changes in the patient population, with new clinical treatments and procedures, and with research. In order to define the structural and procedural changes required to meet these needs, data from activity analyses, ward audits and quality assessments would need to be collected on the current situation in the hospital. Priority options can then be tempered to reflect the availability of finance and nursing skills. If it is to be comprehensive, a nursing strategy will need to consider:

— developments in nursing philosophy and clinical nursing practice needed to satisfy unmet needs.

— environments in which nursing care is delivered and the changes needed for future developments.

— skills typically needed to provide care to different groups of patients at different stages of their illness or hospital stay.

— number and mix of nurses, assistants and support staff needed to provide these skills cost-effectively through the day.

— methods needed to recruit, retain and encourage the return to work of the staff required.

— investment in training, professional and managerial training to ensure that staff are motivated and provide good care.

— necessary changes in management.

— information systems which will help them do this more effectively.

— methods for assessing and improving the quality of patient care and consulting patient opinion.

IMPLEMENTING THE STRATEGY

160. A hospital which has recently implemented extensive changes to staffing, systems and practice on pilot wards found:-

— Good communication with all staff, not just nurses, is essential.

— The backing of the unit policy board and its commitment to providing whatever resources are needed gives credibility with staff.

— The pace and timing of development must be realistic. There are no quick solutions. But some benefits must be visible early on.

— Managing the stress that invariably accompanies major change is important.

— If nurses get personally involved in collecting data about their current activity, they are more likely to be convinced of the need for change.

— Strategies should not be computer driven. Computers are not a substitute for good management.

— Strong leadership is needed.

Conclusion

161. This report has mapped out a broad way forward for managers of ward nursing services, concentrating on areas in which they should take the initiative or where nurses will need their support to effect change and to make a reality of objectives set out in the Patient's Charter. It reflects good practice which already exists in some hospitals. Managers will need to consider how the nursing service can best be developed and managed to match the needs of tomorrow's patients. Management must ensure that a framework for bottom up quality assurance initiatives is in place. They must also develop systems for monitoring patient opinion and quality of care, both through use of appropriate indicators and periodic ward audit. Collective agreement will be required on a strategy for staffing the wards in accordance with measured workload, for support and development of staff and for managing nursing resources. Forthcoming papers will discuss in more detail how some ward sisters are making care more patient centred and improving its continuity within existing budgets and how the best use may be made of the considerable sums now being spent on nurse management systems.

162. During the coming year the Commission's auditors will be reviewing the extent to which efficient and good quality care is given to patients. They will examine strategies for nursing, management structures, the management of human and financial resources, and quality assurance systems. The audit will include a review of the day to day staffing of wards and current and planned ward establishments will be compared with similar wards in other hospitals.

163. A major focus of the audit will be a detailed examination of the organisation of care on the wards, the extent to which care is planned and delivered to patients on an individual rather than a routine basis, and the degree of continuity of care achieved whilst patients are in the hospital. Local auditors will be seeking the views of patients in a survey that uses a questionnaire and a short interview. They will also examine the patients' nursing records. The audit will best be done in partnership with managers and ward based nurses. Wherever possible, health authorities will be asked to attach a nurse to the audit to participate in the review of nursing records. The commitment of senior management will be essential to achieve maximum benefit from the local audits. Pilot audits undertaken so far suggest that this will be readily forthcoming.

SUMMARY OF RECOMMENDATIONS

More large scale research is needed into nursing outcomes and how they are affected both by the number and mix of ward staff and by changes in nursing practice and organisation of care.

1. Delivering Better Patient Care

(i) **QUALITY ASSESSMENT:** Patient opinion surveys should be improved to give more meaningful feedback on specific nursing issues of current relevance. There should be more systematic analysis of themes underlying comment and complaint.

(ii) More use could be made by managers and nurses of indicators such as pressure sore incidence, hospital acquired infection rates, drug errors and patient falls to identify areas for fuller investigation. Quality of care should be assessed regularly and systematically using **simple** packages and results fed back promptly to the wards.

(iii) **QUALITY ASSURANCE:** Management should provide a structure and support for quality assurance initiatives, but nursing standards should be developed by ward staff and address the specific problems of each ward and the care of its patients.

(iv) Management should promote nursing involvement in clinical audit. They should recognise and expand the role of nursing development units in developing and publicising good practice and should agree research and development plans with them.

(v) **MAKING CARE MORE PATIENT CENTRED:** Ward timetables should, as far as is possible, be organised around patients' needs and preferences. Management should monitor this and stimulate change through provision of professional development opportunities. They should facilitate dialogue between nurses and other professions to overcome any obstacles.

(vi) Nurses and managers should show that good care planning matters by giving it adequate priority and time. Managers should ensure that care plans are audited periodically and that sisters allocate responsibility for assessing each individual patient, planning and monitoring his care to a named qualified nurse. Sisters should ensure that decisions about changes to a patient's nursing care are normally made only by that nurse.

(vii) **IMPROVING CONTINUITY OF CARE:** If the spread of primary nursing is to improve care, deep-rooted attitudinal problems need to be addressed first. Those monitoring its implementation should concentrate on the principles of continuity:- the duration of physical allocation of patients to specific nurses, responsibility for decisions and for communication.

(viii) Improved continuity will be dependent on better rostering and more stable ward staffing. Ward sisters' 24 hour responsibility should be matched by control over night staffing. Transfers of patients between wards for non-clinical reasons should be avoided; If essential, more attention should be paid to identifying suitable patients who are willing to move. Managers should ensure that nurses have a 'standard' for ensuring that continuity is maintained.

(ix) Good team nursing may be a better way to promote continuity of care in the short term on wards where staff nurses are as yet unready to take on the additional responsibility of becoming a primary nurse. Nurses should be helped to change their practice through more, and better directed, professional development.

(x) Managers should support initiatives to improve continuity of care such as cutting out intermediaries when the nurses allocated to patients communicate with doctors and others.

(xi)Each unit should have a discharge policy supported by training, monitoring and post-discharge feedback on specific patients. Discharge requirements should be assessed from admission. Managers should provide adequate resources and support for nurses to improve the quality of patient information available on wards.

2. **Staffing the wards**

(i) **EMPLOYING THE 'RIGHT' NUMBERS AND MIX OF STAFF:** Managers should put in place structures to evaluate the effects on care delivery processes, on patient opinion and on staff of all significant changes to ward staffing levels, skill mix and also shift patterns.

(ii) There should be periodic zero-based, *collaborative* review of numbers and skill mix reflecting *agreed* workload for ward to reflect changes to nursing workload and provision of care. Ward activity should first be reviewed and managers should be involved in the review of action plans drawn up by ward sisters to improve efficiency and patient care.

(iii)Workload assessment should be used to inform periodic review of staffing,but the data is more likely to be accurate and cost- effective if it is also of use to nurses on a day-to-day basis.

(iv)Managers should facilitate negotiated change to skill-mix within agreed budgets where nurses consider this desirable to meet patient need. Reviews of support services should include evaluations of the likely effect on the level of non-nursing duties performed by nurses and their cost. Nationally £ 40 millions could be redeployed if best practice in reducing the amount of inappropriate clerical and hosekeeping duties carried out by nurses were replicated.

(v) A co-ordinator should be nominated for implementation of Project 2000 and to communicate decisions affecting the wards.

(vi)**IMPROVING RECRUITMENT & RETENTION:** Managers should make better use of turnover and sickness data to identify potential retention problems in specific areas. Staff views should be surveyed periodically. Exit interviews and questionnaires should be used more systematically to find out why staff leave and to identify measures that might improve retention. Each unit should have a recruitment, retention and return strategy and should set annual targets for improved retention. Individual performance review (IPR) should be extended so that all staff receive adequate feedback on their performance.

(vii) Effective use should be made of the remaining enrolled nurses. Hospital policies which restrict their role and opportunities should be reviewed.

(viii)Personnel departments should provide adequate support for the recruitment of nurses. Greater emphasis should be given to placing each nurse in the most suitable post. If possible, each applicant should be interviewed for several posts. Professional aspects of the induction process should be improved and mentors appointed for new post-holders.

(ix)**DEVELOPING CLINICAL SKILLS:** Managers should provide adequate funding for post-registration education, time for study built into ward establishments and opportunities for cross- fertilisation of ideas with nurses from other wards and hospitals. Nationally it would cost £60 millions to bring *average* levels of post-registration study up to those observed on wards that have adopted primary nursing, but disparities between wards and individual nurses must also be addressed.

(x) Individual performance review (IPR) should be used to identify professional and managerial development needs systematically and to provide data for a balanced post-registration education programme. Continuing training should also be provided for support workers

(xi) **MAKING BEST DAY-TO-DAY USE OF WARD STAFF:** Sisters should be given the education and freedom to negotiate new shift patterns appropriate to ward workload. They should receive help in overcoming barriers to change. In hospitals where there are long afternoon shift overlaps, managers should encourage sisters to review activities during these periods to see whether these could be accommodated more efficiently. Nationally £ 50 millions of nursing resources could be redeployed if overlaps were reduced to 1 hour.

(xii)Training on good rostering which preserves continuity of care should be provided. There should be periodic management audit of the efficiency, effectiveness and equity of rosters.

(xiii)Workload assessment should be concentrated on helping nurses to control and pace their work better. Nurses should be moved from one ward to another only as a last resort, involving ward sisters in the decision.

(xiv)Managers should facilitate agreement between nurses and doctors on those exceptional circumstances when insoluble shortages of nurses over a sustained period would make it advisable in the interests of patients to restrict workload. They should agree the procedures to be followed and methods to be used to reduce workload to levels reflecting nurse availability - restricted admissions, case-mix, transfers, restricted nursing role.

(xv) Flexible rostering agreements should be negotiated as an alternative to excessive employment of bank and agency nurses. Workload assessment and delegated budgets should be used to improve control over the use of temporary staff to 'make up the numbers'.

(xvi) Bank and other temporary nurses should normally be assigned only to wards with which they are familiar. Better induction should be provided for for bank nurses.

3. **Managing the nursing service**
   (i) The role of nursing management should be to develop the service to meet patient needs. Middle managers of nursing should be clinically based. Responsibilities should be clarified.

(ii) Day to day management of staff and budgets should be devolved to wards as far as is possible. Sisters should be given the flexibility to exercise this extended management role positively and the preparation, training and support to do so effectively.

(iii) The objectives of nurse management systems should be clarified and their proposed use 'modelled'. Computerisation of patient information used by nurses should be given priority. Training and support should be directed at improving nurses' awareness of how they can use systems to improve patient care.

(iv) Many hospitals could reduce nurse management costs to 2 per cent of the nursing pay budget without sacrificing quality; nationally this could yield £ 35 millions for redistribution.

(v) Each hospital or unit should have a head of nursing (Matron or DNS) with a seat on the management board to provide professional leadership. She should have responsibility for nursing strategy, practice development and education, but not for day-to-day line management of nurses or nursing budgets.

(vi) A nursing strategy flowing from analysis of patient needs and linked to hospital plans should be developed. Nursing developments should be integrated with those elsewhere so they reflect changes in hospital management and in medical practice.

References

1. V Henderson (1978), The concept of nursing, Journal of Advanced Nursing, 3:113-30

2. Stautory Instrument 873 (1983), Rule 18, under the Nurses, Midwives and Health Visitors Act, HMSO

3. V Beardshaw and R Robinson (1990) New for Old? – Prospects for nursing in the 1990s, King's Fund Institute, London.

4. Nursing Times Editorial (May 1991), Vol 87, No.19

5. The Patient's Charter (1991) and Rt.Hon.John Major - Speech at the Nursing Standard/BUPA Awards Ceremony, 17 September 1991

6. M Calnan and S J Williams (1991), Consumer Satisfaction with Primary, Dental and Hospital Care, University of Kent

7. P J Hibbs (1988), Pressure Area Care, City and Hackney Health Authority

8. B Moores and A G H Thompson (1986), What 1357 hospital inpatients thought about aspects of their stay in British acute hospitals, Journal of Advanced Nursing, 11:87-102

9. Royal College of Surgeons, College of Anaesthetists (1990), Report of the Working Party on Pain After Surgery

10. F E Schmitt amd P J Wooldridge (1973), Psychological preparation of surgical patients, Nursing Research, Vol. 22 2:108-116

11. Department of Health (1961), The Pattern of the In-Patient's Day - Report by a sub-committee of the Standing Nursing Advisory Committee, HMSO

12. S Procter (1989), The functioning of nursing routines in the management of a transient workforce, Journal of Advanced Nursing, 14: 180-189

13. Audit Commission (1992), Lying in Wait – The use of medical beds in acute hospitals, To be published by HMSO shortly

14. J Wilson (1991), Step by painful step, Nursing Times Vol 87, No.38: 42-43

15. H Gaze (1990) Making Time to Talk, Nursing Times Vol 86, No.13: 38-39.

16. Department of Health (1989) Discharge of Patients from Hospital, DoH Circular HC/89/5

17. A Maynard (1987) What Nursing Shortage? Health Service Journal 8/10/1989

18. National Audit Office (1985) National Health Service: Control of Nursing Manpower, HMSO

19. All Wales Nurse Manpower Planning Committee (1987), Third Report -Nursing Staff Mix, Welsh Office

20.J A Ball, K Hurst, M R Booth, R Franklin (1989)'...But Who Will Make the Beds?', Mersey RHA and The Nuffield Institute for Health Services Studies (University of Leeds).

21. NHS Management Consultancy Services/ Nursing Division (1988) Service Quality, Department of Health

22. J Robinson, J Stilwell, C Hawley and N Hempstead (1989), The Role of the Support Worker in the Ward Health Care Team, Nursing Policy Studies 6, University of Warwick

23. A Binnie (1988) Structural Changes, Nursing Times, 83, No.39

24. J Buchan, I Seccombe (1991), Nurse Turnover Costs – A Review for the Royal College of Nursing, Institute of Manpower Studies Report No.212

25. R Waite, J Buchan, J Thomas (1989), Nurses in and out of work, Institute of Manpower Studies Report No.170

26. Mersey RHA Department of Nursing (1989), Job Satisfaction

27. R Waite, G Pike (1989), School Leaver Decline and Effective Local Solutions, Institute of Manpower Studies Report No.178

28. C Todd, N Reid, G Robinson (1990) The Impact of 12-Hour Nursing Shifts, Nursing Times Vol.87, No.31, 47-50.

29. H Orton, D Allsopp (1991) Up Against a Barrier, Health Service Journal 26 September 1991: 28-29

30. M Dehlinger, Nurses' utilization of the computerized record at MIH Clinical Center, in H J Heffernan (ed), Proceedings of the Fifth Annual Symposium on Computer Applications in Medical Care (1990),744-747, IEEE Press, New York.

31. Department of Health Nursing Division (1989) A Strategy for Nursing, HMSO

Appendix 1: CONTACTS AND TEAM MEMBERS

The following NHS hospitals were studied:

— Chesterfield & North Derbyshire Royal Hospital – North Derbyshire HA

— Derriford Hospital – Plymouth HA

— Hinchingbrooke Hospital – Huntingdon HA

— Hope Hospital – Salford HA

— Huddersfield Royal Infirmary – Huddersfield HA

— Kent & Sussex and Pembury Hospitals – Tunbridge Wells HA

— Prince Phillip Hospital, Llanelli – East Dyfed HA

— St Mary's and Queen Alexandra Hospitals – Portsmouth HA

— Westminster Hospital – Riverside HA

— Weymouth & District Hospital – West Dorset HA

Briefer study visits were paid to:

— Bury HA (Fairfield General Hospital)

— Freeman Hospital, Newcastle upon Tyne

— Homerton Hospital (City & Hackney HA)

— Queen Mary's Hospital, Roehampton

— Princess Grace Hospital, London – AMI Group

— West Middlesex University Hospital

— Ysbyty Glan Clwyd

— Ysbyty Gwynedd, Bangor

The following French and American Hospitals were also studied:

— Beth Israel Hospital, Boston, Massachusets, USA

— Fairfax Hospital, Falls Church, Virginia, USA

— Strong Memorial Hospital, Rochester, New York, USA

— Hotel Dieu de Paris

— Hopital du Mans

— Ecole des Cadres, Paris

Thanks are due to colleagues in the United States (OIG), France (IGAS) and Sweden (SPRI) for arranging visits and supplying information.

The interdisciplinary team which conducted the study comprised

— Jocelyn Cornwell

— Ian Jones

— David Shepherd

— Eileen Shepherd (RGN, Dip.N)

— Ken Sneath
  and was assisted by Andy Tighe

The members of the Project Advisory Group were:

— Jean Ball, Nuffield Institute for Health Studies

— Heather Cawthorne, Department of Health Nursing Division [*]

— Alison Kitson, Institute of Nursing, Radcliffe Infirmary and Director of the RCN Standards
  of Care Project

— Helen Quinn, Nuffield Institute for Health Studies
  (formerly Regional Project Nurse, Northern RHA)

— Jane Robinson, Professor of Nursing, Nottingham University Medical School

— Jane Salvage, Regional Director for Europe (Nursing), WHO
  (formerly Director of Nursing Developments, Kings Fund)

— Caroline Storey, Regional Project Nurse, South Western RHA

— Bert Telford, Director of Operations, Burton-on-Trent DGH.

— Kevin Woods, Regional Planning Officer, Trent RHA
  (formerly District General Manager, Chester DHA)

The project team was also advised by a group of ward sisters and nurse managers:

— Sue Cooper, Ward Sister, Kent & Sussex Hospital

— Glen Smith, Nursing Officer (Medical Directorate), Chesterfield & North Derbyshire Royal
  Hospital

— Thelma Waters, Divisional Nurse Manager (Surgical Services), Hinchingbrooke Hospital

— Wendy Wild, Ward Sister, St Mary's Hospital, Portsmouth

  Eileen Shepherd, Senior Sister, Health Care of the Elderly, City Hospital Unit, Nottingham
  (formerly of West Middlesex University Hospital) acted as a consultant to the team.

---

[*]   *Heather Cawthorne replaced Sue Norman, Department of Health, who attended the first two meetings of the advisory
      group.*

The following regional nurses were consulted or offered comments on earlier drafts of the report:

— Rosemary Knights, Regional Nursing Officer, Mersey RHA

— Sheila Roy, Regional Nursing Officer, North West Thames RHA

— Susan Cowie, Nurse Manpower Project, North Western RHA

— Margaret Farrington-Wood, Mersey RHA

— Una McDonnell, Mersey RHA

— Jill Pooley, Trent RHA

Advice was recieved from many others including:

— Adrian Bagust, Health Economics Consortium, University of York (formerly NWRHA)

— Alison Binnie, Senior Sister, John Radcliffe Hospital, Oxford

— John Birch, North Lincolnshire HA

— Nick Black and Colleagues
at the London School of Hygiene and Tropical Medicine

— Meg Bond, University of Warwick

— Senga Bond, University of Newcastle

— Jim Buchan, Institute of Manpower Studies, University of Sussex

— Roy Carr-Hill and Colleagues
at the Centre for Health Economics, University of York

— Christine Hancock, General Secretary, Royal College of Nursing

— Alan Hislop, Directorate of Health Service Information Systems, Edinburgh

— Jennifer Hunt, Chief Nurse Adviser, Royal Brompton Hospital

— Ken Jarrold, Regional General Manager, Wessex

— Anne McPherson, Director of Quality & Nursing Development, East Hertfordshire HA

— Jillian Maguire, University Hospital of Wales, Cardiff

— Gloria Oates, District General Manager, Rochdale HA

— Susan Proctor, Newcastle Polytechnic

— Diana Sale, formerly Nursing Adviser to West Dorset HA

— Andy Thompson, Cardiff University Business School

— Richard Waite, formerly Institute of Manpower Studies,
University of Sussex

— Shirley Williams, Oxford Community Unit

— Jo Wilson, Senior Nurse, Freeman Hospital, Newcastle

71

The following organisations were consulted during the study or commented on the report in draft:

— Association of Community Health Councils

— Confederation of Health Service Employees (COHSE)

— Conference of Royal Colleges

— Department of Health

— English National Board

— Institute of Health Service Management

— National Association of Health Authorities and Trusts

— National Union of Public Employees (NUPE)

— NHS Trusts Federation

— Patients' Association

— Royal College of Nursing (RCN)

— Scottish Home and Health Department

— Trades Union Congress

— United Kingdom Central Council for Nursing, Midwifery and Health Visitors (UKCC)

— Welsh National Board

— Welsh Office

Appendix 2: GLOSSARY

Accreditation

Periodic inspection of structure and process of services relevant to hospital patient care against specified criteria and standards, providing a certificate of approval. Mandatory in USA, Canada, Australia etc. In the UK the King's Fund has piloted a voluntary package.

Acuity

The average dependency of patients on a ward. (But sometimes used synonymously with dependency or nursing workload).

Acute Wards

Wards caring for emergency or elective inpatients with severe symptoms whilst they are undergoing short term treatment or investigation.

Agency Nurse

A temporary nurse booked through a commercial agency supplying staff to hospitals, nursing homes etc.

Assessment

The process of gathering and evaluating information about the patient's health status, home and personal circumstances on admission to the ward in order that nursing problems can be identified and a holistic nursing care plan formulated.

Associate nurse

Nurse in a ward practising 'primary nursing' who cares for specific patients when the 'primary nurse' with 24 hour responsibility for planning and directing care given to those patients is off duty. An associate nurse may also have her own primary caseload, but in the UK is more likely to be a junior nurse or learner who supports a particular primary nurse.

Auxiliary

An unqualified member of the ward team, contributing to straightforward aspects of the direct care of suitable patients under the supervision of a (qualified) nurse.

Bank Nurse

A temporary nurse supplied to a ward from a list maintained by the hospital or unit of part-time staff willing to work specified hours on nominated days.

Care Plan

Prioritised plan of nursing care to be provided to an individual patient whilst in hospital,based on problems identified during the assessment and preferably drawn up in consultation with the patient or relations. Progress should be evaluated against goals on review dates specified in the plan. Standardised pre-printed care plans are frequently used for short stay surgical patients.

Case Management (in the Acute Hospital setting)

Interdisciplinary model of patient care involving formulation of an agreed 'care map' for groups of patients with similar diagnoses, appointment of a case manager (usually a nurse) to plan and progress the care and discharge of those patients,and systematic analysis of reasons for deviance from the care map. The care map replaces the care plan, usually allowing limited individualisation.

Charge nurse

Male equivalent to a ward sister.

Clinical Grading

Career progression ladder for nurses (A-I) linked to responsibilities and qualification introduced in 1988.

73

Clinical Tutor	A teacher from the College of Nursing who provides clinical training and support to student nurses during ward placements. A disappearing breed.
Conversion Course	Course for enrolled nurses wishing to convert to registered nurse status.
Criteria for Care	A widespread dependency based workload assessment methodology, including periodic activity analysis, usually linked to the MONITOR quality assessment package.
Cyclical Roster	An off duty roster which repeats after a standard period rather than being drawn up individually each fortnight or month.
Dependency	An assessment of a patient's ability to care for himself, eg with regard to feeding, personal hygiene and mobility. A broader definition is sometimes used embracing the patient's total need for nursing care including education, rehabilitation and psychological care.
Discharge Plan	A plan, based on an assessment of the patient's home circumstances and abilities, of action needed to prepare for satisfactory discharge and to put in place any services or aids that he will need if he is to care for himself at home.
District Nursing Advisor (DNA) District Nursing Officer (DNO)	Chief Nurse providing professional nursing advice to the District Executive, – the line management DNO post has in general disappeared with the Reforms.
Director of Nursing Services (DNS)	Chief Nurse within a Hospital or Unit, not necessarily with line management responsibilities for nurses.
Drug Rounds	Ward rounds at specified times, normally between 5 and 8 times a day in general wards, to dispense prescribed drugs.
Dynamic Standard Setting System (DySSSy)	The Royal College of Nursing Standards of Care Project. A structure and methodology for nursing quality assurance involving the setting, monitoring and reassessment of ward based standards.
Early Shift	The first daytime shift, typically from around 07.30 to 15.30.
English National Board (ENB)	The validating and examining body for nurse, midwife and health visitor training and education in England.
Enrolled Nurse (EN)	A 'second level' practical nurse qualified, after 2 years training, through enrolment to the nurses' register. Graded C, D, exceptionally E.
Evaluation	Appraisal, against a set of criteria, of the effectiveness of the nursing care delivered to a patient in achieving specified goals. The evaluation may show that his care plan needs to be changed or updated.
First Level Nurse	Registered nurse (q.v.).
Float	Nursing Pool (q.v.)
Funded Establishment	The number of staff at each grade funded in the budget for the ward or unit.

Handover	Procedure whereby nurses going off duty hand over responsibility for patient care to the new shift, telling them key facts about each patient; eg: impending treatment, changes in condition or care.
Health Care Assistant (HCA) Health Care Support Worker (HCSW)	Support staff, with locally determined pay and conditions, recruited on implementation of P2000 to replace the traditional learner service contribution. Role varies according to setting but may include elements of direct patient care, clerical and housekeeping duties. Training leading to eventually 4 levels of NVQ is promised.
'Heavy End'	Colloquial term for the area of award to which patients in a more stable condition, but requiring a lot of lifting and predominantly non-technical nursing care (eg stroke victims), are allocated. (Such segregation is not advocated if avoidable).
Holistic Care	Care directed at meeting all of the patient's physical, emotional, social and spiritual needs as an integrated whole, rather than treating each problem or disease separately.
Home Assessment	Visit by an occupational– and/or physio-therapist, social worker or home care organiser, possibly accompanied by a primary nurse, to the patient's home prior to discharge to assess the need for support services, adaptations and installation of aids to mobility.
ICU / ITU	Intensive Care/Therapy Unit housing patients requiring ventilation, 24 hour observation and specialist nursing care on a 1:2 or 1:1 basis.
Individualised Patient Care(IPC)	Conceptual approach to provision of holistic care over the period of a patient's stay based on an assessment of each patient's individual care needs.
Individual Performance Review (IPR)	Staff appraisal system involving evaluation of performance against specific individually agreed objectives and identification of development needs.
Internal Rotation	Shift pattern whereby all (or most) ward staff take turns to provide night-time cover, so abolishing or reducing the separate night nursing staff.
Junior Sister	Deputy to the ward sister (grade 'F').
'Kardex'	Term still commonly used for part of each patient's nursing record, summarising admission information and providing a continuation record.
Late (shift)	The second daytime shift, typically from around 14.30 to 21.30.
Learner	Student or pupil nurse on traditional (apprenticeship style) course.
Liaison Nurse	Nurse responsible for liaising between hospital and community nurses about arrangements for the continuing care of specified patients.
Long Day (shift)	Shift covering part of the late shift as well as the morning. (In some hospitals a 12 hour long day shift is worked).
Magnet Hospital (USA)	Hospital which by adopting an innovative style of nursing and good management practices is able to attract and retain high quality nursing staff.
Matron	This former title for the chief nurse in a hospital is undergoing a revival.

Mentor	Nurse nominated to teach, oversee and support a student nurse during a ward placement.
Model (of Nursing)	A conceptual framework for nursing practice, embodying knowledge, beliefs and values, adopted by a ward or unit as the basis of a common direction and ethos. The most common theoretical models in use on general wards are Orem's self care model and Roper's Activities of Living model. The term is also sometimes used to describe the chosen form of organisation of care (eg Primary Nursing).
MONITOR	A quality assessment tool used to evaluate the ward environment and the process of care (including patient documentation).
Nurse Management System	Computerised system assisting the management of nursing through workload assessment (sometimes linked to care planning), rostering, analysis of staff costs, retrieval of personnel data etc.
Nursing Audit	Systematic procedure for assessment and discussion nursing care delivered to specific categories of patients on one or more wards with a view to evaluating effectiveness and ethical desirability of elements of that care.
Nursing Development Unit (NDU)	Ward (or other unit) granted supplementary funding (eg through the King's Fund) to implement, evaluate and publicise an agreed programme of clinical development.
Nursing Process	A systematic problem solving approach to patient centred nursing care, nominally adopted throughout the UK in the 1980s. The aim is to prevent, alleviate or minimise 'problems' presented by the individual patient. Components of the process are 'assessment', formulation of a 'care plan', its 'implementation' and 'evaluation' of the outcomes.
Off-duty	Nursing shift roster or schedule.
On Take	Periods when a ward is the planned destination for emergency admissions.
Organisation of care	The method by which nurses and auxiliaries are allocated to patients or given care tasks on a day to day basis (e.g. Patient Allocation, Team Nursing)
Outliers	Patients who, because of pressure on bed or staff availability, are housed on a ward inappropriate for their condition.
Overlap	Period (early afternoon in particular) when more than one shift is on duty.
Patient Allocation	Method of organising care whereby each patient is allocated one or more nurses for the duration of a shift.
Patient Centred Care	Individualised, holistic care dictated by the needs and wishes of each patient rather than by the values or convenience of nurses.
Patient Education	Explanation and advice given to patients to enable them to cope with any disability, assist discharge and prevent avoidable readmission to hospital.
Pool	Central pool of nurses and auxiliaries within a hospital available for allocation to short-staffed wards.
Preceptor	Nurse allocated to help and advise an inexperienced member of staff.

PREPP	The UKCC's proposed Post-Registration Education and Practice Project, currently at the consultative stage. It would require all registered nurses to undertake at least 5 days continuing professional education every 3 years to remain on the Register.
Pressure area care	Action to prevent or treat bed sores in non-ambulant patients.
Primary Nursing	Nursing philosophy and organisation of care whereby the 'primary nurse', nominated for each patient on admission, assumes 24 hour responsibility and authority for all aspects of that patient's nursing care during his stay.
Project 2000	Initiative to replace traditional 'apprenticeship' style pre-registration training for nurses and make consequent changes to ward staffing. An 18 month college based core programme is followed by a specialist 'branch'. Students receive grants instead of salaries and are supernumerary during ward experience placements, being replaced by HCAs.
Pupil Nurse	Student on a 2 year enrolled nurse course. (Virtually obsolete).
Quality Assessment	Measurement of quality of the ward environment, nursing documentation and delivery of care, eg using a preformulated tool such as MONITOR.
Quality Assurance	Process of defining problems in care delivery, implementing measures to overcome them, measuring the results and reassessing the need for further action.
Registered General Nurse (RGN)	A qualified nurse who has completed a 3 year course of training and is on the UKCC's General Register. Other types of registered nurse are RMNs (Psychiatric) RSCN (Children), RNMS (Mental Handicap).
Rostering	Allocation of shift duties to ward staff.
Royal College of Nursing (RCN)	Professional body for nursing and trade union.
Skill mix	The percentage of ward staff who are qualified. Or, more broadly, the mix of nursing skills possessed by ward staff, for example on a particular shift.
Staff Nurse (SN)	A permanently employed registered nurse, usually graded D or E.
Standards	Statements of the levels of service or care related to specific topics which ward staff agree to provide. Normally accompanied by a description of the structure (staff, equipment etc) and process needed to attain specified observable (preferably quantified) outcomes. See also 'DySSSy'.
Supernumerary	Nurses (eg P2000 students) who are not included in the funded establishment and who are not assumed to make a specific contribution to patient care.
Second Level Nurse	Enrolled nurse (q.v.).
Take day	Day when a ward is "On Take" (q.v.).
Task Allocation	Method of organising care whereby each specific type of care is carried out by a separate nominated nurse.

Team Nursing	Method of organising care based on allocation of each nurse to a team which cares for a group of patients for a number of shifts. (nb: used differently in the American literature).
Telford	A frequently used consultative establishment setting methodology.
Time Out	Analysis of time spent by nursing staff away from the wards: sick, on leave, studying, or for example escorting patients or on other non ward duties.
TPRs	Nursing abbreviation for the recording of a patient's temperature, blood pressure and respiration.
United Kingdom Central Council for Nursing, Midwifery and Health Visitors (UKCC)	The professional registration and disciplinary body for all nurses in the United Kingdom.
Ward Clerk	Assistant, often part time, based on a ward primarily to obtain and file medical records, undertake routine clerical duties, answer the telephone and deal with straightforward enquiries.
Ward Co-ordinator	Modern title of role replacing that of 'nurse in charge' of a shift, commonly used on wards practising primary nursing.
Ward Domestic or Ward Orderly	Person primarily providing cleaning services to the ward.
Ward Manager	Modern title for the person in overall charge of a ward. i.e. Either the ward sister/charge nurse (especially on those primary nursing wards where the ward manager does not retain a major direct patient care role) or, exceptionally, a non-nurse employed to manage and co-ordinate ward staff.
Ward Philosophy	A statement in plain language drawn up by ward nurses of the aims of patient care on their ward. It should be specific to that ward and to the types of patients normally treated on it.
Ward Sister	Nurse responsible for the management and development of a ward and its staff and for ensuring the standards of care which they provide. (Grade G, or exceptionally H or I for Senior Sisters with additional management responsibilities beyond the ward).
Welsh National Board (WNB)	The validating and examining body for nurse, midwife and health visitor training and education in Wales.
Whole time equivalent (wte)	Total weekly contracted hours of full and part time staff expressed as a multiple of the standard working week (37.5 hours).